D0859105

The Victim

Is Always

the Same

THE VICTIM

IS ALWAYS

THE SAME

I. S. Cooper, M.D.

The Norton Library

W·W·NORTON & COMPANY·INC·

NEW YORK

Copyright © 1973 by I. S. Cooper. All rights reserved. Published simultaneously in
Canada by George J. McLeod Limited, Toronto. Printed in the United States of America.
First published in the Norton Library 1976 by arrangement with Harper & Row,
Publishers, Inc.

Books That Live
The Norton imprint on a book means that in the publisher's
estimation it is a book not for a single season but for the years.
W. W. Norton & Company, Inc.

The quotation on page xxi is from *Resistance, Rebellion and Death* by Albert Camus,
translated by Justin O'Brien. Copyright ® 1960 by Alred A. Knopf, Inc. Reprinted by
permission of the publisher.

The photographs on pages 134, 137, 139 by Henry Groskinsky originally appeared in *Life*
Magazine, © 1972 Time Inc. All other photographs were taken by Rosemary Spitaleri.
Drawings were done by Mary Lorenc.

The names of the staff members of St. Barnabas Hospital are real, but the names of the
patients have been changed.

Library of Congress Cataloging in Publication Data

Cooper, Irving Spencer, 1922-
    The victim is always the same.

    (The Norton Library)
    Reprint of the ed. published by Harper & Row, New York.
    1. Brain—Surgery.   2.   Dystonia musculorum deformans.
3. Children—Surgery.   4.   Medical ethics.   I.   Title.
RD594.C66   1976   617'.481   76-12485
ISBN 0-393-00817-7

1 2 3 4 5 6 7 8 9 0

DEDICATION TO

Sissel

Dan, Doug, Lisa, and David

WHOM I LOVE

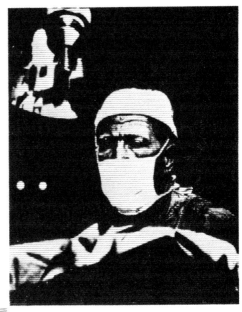

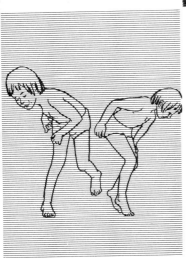

Foreword

This is an unusual book. It is an unexpected book. It is extremely readable. The author, who is world-famed for his originality and technical skill as a surgeon has given us evidence of something much more. These pages reveal his serious thinking and his great humanity.

The reader will find three distinct topics, each one of which is likely to fascinate. The writer starts, and finishes, by thoughtful essays on some of the ethical problems which more and more confront medical practitioners in their handling of sick persons who have blindly entrusted to them their health and lives. The topical problems are currently exercising the conscience of the medical profession throughout the world. Doctors are still debating these issues and, to date, no rigid rulings have emerged. Dr. Cooper's contribution is all the more important on that account, for it will provoke constructive thinking.

A series of chapters deal with the case histories of two young children who had insidiously developed that most distressing and grotesque of maladies, dystonia musculorum. Dr. Cooper tells us how his interest in this fantastic affliction was aroused when, as a young naval surgeon, he made a post-graduate visit to Montefiore Hospital in New York. What he saw of the victims coiling and writhing in uncontrollable spasms impressed him so deeply that they became etched into his memory as a distressing image. This malady, rare enough in the United States, is a clinical curiosity in Great Britain. This writer, too, can vividly recall the impact and shock when a visiting neurologist from the same Montefiore Hospital came to London in 1925 and showed films of these patients to an astonished audience. The earliest stages of this affliction are mild and the progression stealthy. Indeed in the early stages the symptoms may be inconsistent. It is not surprising that the suspicion that the disability is not an organic one can be legitimately entertained for a while. There is no excuse, however, for persisting obstinately in this error, and a note of horror is struck as one reads of the tribulations of Susan and Janet until they eventually received the correct diagnostic appraisal at the hands of neurologists who were belatedly consulted. One likes to think that such a fate could never again befall these victims.

Dr. Cooper then reveals to us the story of the origins of the current practice of cryothalamectomy: how it arose as a fragment of serendipity, shrewdly perceived and assessed and then cautiously repeated as an empirical gesture which seemed promising. He leads us into the wards of his hospital and allows us to listen to the gentleness of his handling of the hostile and tortured victims and of their distressed parents who had reached their tether's end. Then Dr. Cooper conducts us into the operating theater of St. Barnabas Hospital and reveals to us in simple language the successive stages of the operative ritual. We witness a miracle of technical skill and patience, coupled with infinite courage and confidence on the part of the patient, who may have to submit to two, three or even more brain operations before a restitution to normalcy is achieved. The end results are at times so considerable as to astound even an experienced neurologist with his memories of the failures of conventional drug therapy, physical medicine, and psychiatric assaults in this most humiliating and crippling of afflictions.

This book is not written primarily for a medical reader, although some of the chapters are founded upon addresses given to professional audiences. Few doctors, however, can fail to be intrigued, and not many will be able to lay it aside without reading it from beginning to end in a single sitting.

Macdonald Critchley, C.B.E., M.C., F.R.C.P.
President, World Federation of Neurology

London
November, 1972

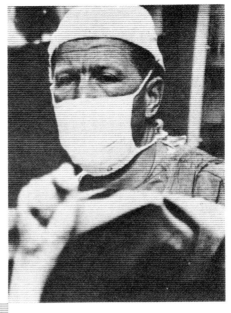

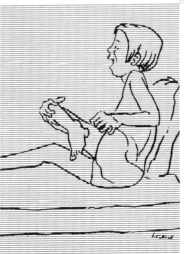

Preface

In 1965 I was invited by the *Mayo Clinic Alumnus Review* to prepare an essay that discussed the moral and ethical principles that should guide clinical investigations involving patients.

In that piece, "Medicine of the Absurd," I spoke of the basic fact that the individual exists in his most naked, lonely, anxious, defenseless state when he is ill and hospitalized. Although he is faced with more acute questions and is more immediately confronted by the filamentous line between Being and Nonbeing, he is at the same time increasingly surrounded by a faceless technology that separates him from the outside.

Hope often seems remote, while at the same time previously abstract considerations of life, death, and dying become concrete.

For the most part, our culture and education has estranged us from confronting such matters as the purpose of life. This has been particularly true of those like ourselves in the medical profession, who must be continually educated in the scientific and technologic aspects of our applied art—an art which forces one to fragment human problems and human beings in the pursuit of his calling.

In dealing with illness, the human condition in its most stark and solitary state, our education has trained us to witness human suffering analytically and to be detached. Sometimes, however, as Henry Knowles Beecher, Distinguished Professor of Anesthesiology at Harvard University, has pointed out, investigations have allowed their detachment from human values to become indifferent. Or, as Ray Herbert Bixler, Professor of Psychology at the University of Louisville in Kentucky, has stated, the analytic stance may become one of arrogance, confusing technique as an end rather than a means.

In my view, when this occurs, the goal of medicine—to make sick people well, or failing that, to relieve pain and suffering—becomes obscured. If this goal is lost sight of—through overfragmentation or arrogance, or failure to realize that man is the end—medicine and medical research then become out of harmony with reason.

Moreover, this cultural evisceration or dehumanization has widened the gulf between lawyers and clients, clergymen and parishioners, artists and subjects, teachers and students, and particularly between humanists, in the classical sense, and humans. Even the modern novel, like modern painting, has become fragmented, as the technique has become an end rather than a means. As though art could have a meaning apart from humanity.

I have chosen medicine as my example because, in my opinion, it stands closest to the union of scientific and humane values; either these fuse harmoniously in medicine or medicine becomes absurd. I have chosen medicine because I have, over two decades, had to enter into the suffering of thousands of individuals—each facing his mortal question alone, each no longer free, each a victim without having done anything wrong, each a microcosmic but magnified view of the tragic human condition.

The anguish caused by fragmentation and analysis is a human problem. It can be ameliorated only by humans—physicians, philosophers, artists, among others, acting humanely—even though ultimate questions remain unanswered.

I have attempted, from my own experience, to record the struggle of two children, twisted and tortured through no fault of their own, to enter the human world of being and time.

This book deals with the anguish and courage of two young girls, Janet and Susan. Although part of their story is concerned with a type of brain surgery, the subject of brain surgery is incidental to the theme. I purposely selected these two children, more disabled than most with the same affliction, in whom the ultimate effect of surgery is not yet determined, so that the remaining fragility of each of them would be central to their trial. The failure or success of a particular therapeutic method, or specialty or technique, is not actually germane.

I could not hope to convey their human condition adequately in words. I should have wished to write a poem had I been able, for perhaps in poetry one could compress the strength, maturity, courage, loneliness, torment, despair, effort, faith, humanity of these children. In their condition is the distillate of human authenticity. In spite of the condition inflicted upon them, they remain loyal to life and to themselves.

What these children—each patient—each person—each

human problem urgently requires is for each of us to return, however difficult it may be, to questions of ultimate concern. Some of the specific questions are confronted in the last chapter. They are starkly implicit in Janet's story. Janet's encounter with nothingness is our own.

There is a natural sense of difference, and as William Barrett points out in his book, *Time of Need: Forms of Imagination in the Twentieth Century,* a feeling of superiority that the living feel toward the dead. This extends to a similar feeling of the strong for the weak and the well for the ill. In the latter instance, it is wrong. Though victims, Janet and Susan were superior, stronger, and wiser than those about them.

Doctors, psychologists, scientists, humanists—even political leaders—seeking after information often fail to look where it is happening. These children speak to us from a region of a happening that others have only wondered or speculated about. They have lived part way over the border between humanity and nothingness. In this region in between, they have found a vast expanse of inhumanity, where it need not exist. It is their message I have tried to carry.

This message is, I hope, implicit in their story. It deals principally with dehumanization—the treatment of people as objects in an increasingly technologic world—and suggests some reasonable approaches to the problem. I should like to state without qualification that an indictment of psychiatry and the behavioral sciences is neither intended nor implied. In certain instances, which are cited, this discipline was abused. This is sometimes true of other disciplines as well—my own included. The developing behavioral sciences, however, now and in the future, are among the great comforts and hopes of mankind. Anyone interpreting the events described as a general criticism of psychiatry would be in error. Sigmund Freud once wrote that the great weakness of psychoanalysis was that it lay beyond human capability. Perhaps the cases cited here bear out Freud's fears of this kind of subjective approach to his art.

When anyone brings up the slave in the colonies and calls for justice, he is reminded of prisoners in Russian concentration camps, and vice versa. And if you protest against the assassination in Prague of an opposition historian like Kalandra, two or three American Negroes are thrown in your face. In such a disgusting attempt at outbidding, one thing only does not change—the victim, prostituted—freedom —and then we notice that everywhere, together with freedom, justice is also profaned.

—ALBERT CAMUS
from "Bread and Freedom,"
Resistance, Rebellion, and Death

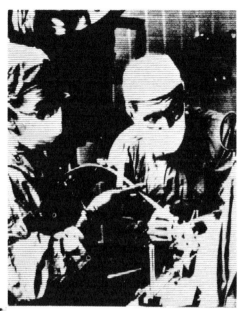

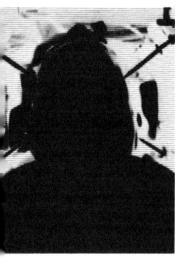

CHAPTER 1

His team of nurses, technicians, and surgical residents were already scrubbed and dressed, cap to pants, in green. The cryotechnician held up for inspection a slender, stainless-steel tube, ten inches long and only one-eighth of an inch in diameter. The tube was the cryoprobe, a slim, hollow, surgical instrument whose tip could be refrigerated to temperatures far below freezing. This instrument would be introduced into the waiting child's brain, and the resident examined it to be certain that it was absolutely straight, that it had not been bent or damaged during the sterilization process.

John Orzuchowski, the cryotechnician, his huge frame exaggerated by the bulky green scrub suit, carefully adjusted the dials on a large white console—the heart of the freezing surgical system. During the operation, Orzuchowski's manipulation of these dials would control the flow of liquid nitrogen, and the oozing fluid whose temperature is 196 degrees centigrade below zero, would flow into the cannula and to the freezing tip of the cryoprobe.

Peg Ryan, whose skilled, gloved hands had assisted the surgeon thousands of times during the past fifteen years, aligned the retractible V-shaped arm that held the flexible conduit, through which the refrigerating liquid nitrogen flowed from its container in the console to the sensitive probe, which the surgeon would use as a frozen scalpel.

Since their first operation together in September 1954, she had assisted him in the performance of more operations on the human brain than any other scrub nurse who ever lived. But today, like the surgeon, she was tense, alert, silently but overwhelmingly conscious of their difficult task and particularly of the frightened child who was the ultimate center of their concern.

The child lay there, in the middle of the gleaming, tiled room, appearing lost on the large operating table, an eleven-year-old girl. Her tiny head was newly shaved and about to be placed in the viselike grip of the special head-holder on the operating table. This headholder—four upright steel beams attached to the upper end of the table—encased the patient's head like the four corners of a square box with its sides open. From each beam a slender, pointed

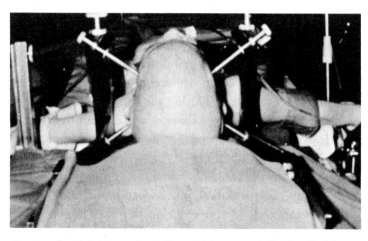

Her tiny head held steady in the viselike grip of the headholder on the operating table, her thin arms spastically extended. Awake, helpless, frightened, lonely, brave, desperately hopeful. Eleven years old.

clamp attached to the child's skull in order to hold it absolutely immobile during the operative procedure. Once the head is fixed and unable to move because of these clamps, even though the limbs and body might writhe involuntarily, the cranium and its precious contents remain fixed and its position constant. Thus the accuracy and safety of the probe placement within the brain, which is measured within fractions of an inch, is made possible.

Her disease (dystonia musculorum deformans) continued to twist and contort her body uncontrollably. The surgeon would soon gently place his probe deep within a small part of her brain, the thalamus. There, in an attempt to relieve the involuntary movements that racked her young body, he would freeze and destroy a hidden group of cells.

She lay there: wide-eyed, tear-stained, frightened. Head shaven, helpless, ignominious in her own view, she was held to the table by the minuscule clamps that adhered to the sides of her head. Feeling nothing, everything, unbelieving, but most of all, feeling alone.

That day in May of 1971 was gray, cloudy, and rainy. The decaying rooftops were visible through the windows of the scrub-up room, which was located between the two neurosurgical operating rooms on the sixth floor of St. Barnabas Hospital in the Bronx. At 8:30, the surgeon was alone at the sinks, pHisohexing his hands and arms to an inch or two above the elbow.

As the surgeon scrubbed, his glance rested on the rooftops which obscured Montefiore Hospital. The first time he'd ever seen a case of dystonia musculorum deformans was in that hospital in the spring of 1945, twenty-six years ago. He had graduated from George Washington

University School of Medicine only a few months before. While serving his internship at the United States Naval Hospital at St. Albans in Queens, he and several of his colleagues had traveled one day that spring across the same Long Island Sound that stretched beyond the window through which he now looked. They had come to Montefiore Hospital to follow along on the teaching rounds of a famous neurologist there.

The young intern was already planning to make a career of neurology and neurosurgery. What had led him to choose this field was the fact that in his freshman year at medical school, when introduced to neuroanatomy, he fell in love with the brain. He loved what appeared to be the logic of the various nervous pathways and of the sensations coming into the nervous system through a specific receptor and going along certain pathways and being interpreted in the brain, which, in turn, controlled the person, and which in the end made him a complex, individual personality. The profundity of the organ, the fact that life really existed in the brain, soon became apparent to him: you are your brain and vice versa. People now talk about the possibility of brain transplant, but if one could really transplant a brain, what he'd be doing instead is transplanting a body around the brain, for all of one's thoughts, one's memories, and one's personality are in the brain and nowhere else. His interest in this master organ, perhaps the unique mystery and challenge in our universe, led to his early decision to pursue the neurologic sciences, and if possible, to become a brain surgeon when his navy internship and service were behind him.

But that morning he was shaken by the grotesque human tragedy he saw in the ward that contained a dozen or more children and young adults with advanced cases of dystonia musculorum deformans. The ward was long and yellowish-gray. Each steel bed with its prison bar head and foot rails contained a contorted mobile of condensed suffering. These were patients with legs and arms pretzel-twisted, backs superbent—some convex, some concave—necks twisted so that the head could not bring its eyes in line to witness its own helplessness, the only movements involuntary, painful spasms or tremors. Walking along behind the professor and looking at these suffering people, the embryo surgeon asked himself, "My God, what is it—this dystonia—that it can do such terrible, degrading things to human beings?"

This affliction, one of the most cruel and intractable scourges of the central nervous system, was described about the same time by Dr. H. L. Parker, a neurologist at the Mayo Clinic:

There is no known treatment of any value for this spasmodic disease affecting muscles. . . . As seen in spasmodic torticollis, the whole neck has to be paralyzed in order to stop its involuntary motion, and to hang like that of a dead fowl in the meat market. A therapeutic result is thereby obtained which is not gladly suffered or gratefully received by the patient or his relatives. . . . In the final and long drawn-out stages over many years, the patient sooner or later becomes bedfast. Contractures have developed and the spasms still try feebly to work on joints fixed beyond repair. It is then that the patient dies from bedsores and inanition. It is, in truth, not a pleasant disease, and possibly in the end, death is welcomed gladly.*

This abysmal view of the therapeutic possibilities for

* H. L. Parker, *Clinical Studies in Neurology* (Charles C Thomas, Springfield, Ill., 1956).

7

dystonia musculorum deformans, so succinctly summarized by Dr. Parker, first became known to the surgeon that day in the spring of 1945. The rows of beds filled with deformed, incapacitated bodies, provided overwhelming evidence that Dr. Parker was right. In the absence of any therapeutic possibility at that time, death would have indeed been welcomed by most of the victims of the disease.

Six years later, in the spring of 1951, he had completed his training in neurosurgery at the Mayo Clinic and had come to teach and practice at the medical school of New York University, University Hospital. During the next two years, while carrying out an investigation of various types of involuntary movement disorders in humans, he had serendipitously discovered that a new and seemingly radical type of brain surgery could reverse the involuntary movements and abnormal postures of dystonia.

In October of 1951, a forty-year-old truck driver from Philadelphia came to the neurosurgical clinic at the University Hospital, seeking some kind of relief for an uncontrollable shaking of his right side. His symptom had started ten years before and had gradually increased to such severity that he could no longer work or use his right hand to feed himself, and was essentially incapacitated in his activities of daily living. After he had been studied by the clinic staff, a decision was made to offer a surgical treatment that might control the shaking to some degree. However, the operation carried a great risk because relief of the tremor was provided by means of sacrificing motor power of the arm and leg, that is, actually producing a partial paralysis of the right side. A high price to pay for relief of the shaking, but one which the patient readily accepted if only he could have some surcease from the constant involuntary movements that racked him.

Throughout the first half of this century, surgeons had sought some means to relieve involuntary movements by operating on the brain. They were stimulated to do so because up to that time there was no successful medical therapy for these symptoms. The most common involuntary movements were those due to Parkinsonism, or "the shaking palsy," a million victims of which existed in the United States alone. However, many other afflictions of the central nervous system produced bizarre, contorting involuntary movements, and the incapacitation as well as the social embarrassment led many of its victims to submit to investigative brain operations in some hope of achieving relief from their symptoms.

At the turn of the century, Sir Victor Horsley, the father of modern brain surgery, operating in England, removed part of the cerebral cortex from the surface of the brain in several patients who had involuntary movements. He reported that by removing that portion of the cerebral cortex, which principally controlled motor activity of the arm and leg on the opposite side of the body, he could achieve some relief of the involuntary movements while lessening the patient's ability to perform voluntary movements at the same time. Years later, neurosurgeons in this country approached the problem following Horsley's lead. A prodigious worker in this field was Paul Bucy of Chicago, who carried out operations similar to those performed by Horsley, and who reported that by inducing partial paralysis in limbs that trembled, the tremors could be relieved, although some loss of motor power appeared inevitable.

Professor Bucy's work was followed by that of Tracy Putnam of the Neurological Institute of New York, who cut fibers in the spinal cord, which descends from the motor cortex in the so-called pyramidal or motor tract. His results were essentially the same: the tremor could be relieved, but motor power often had to be sacrificed. However, the ability to use the arm and leg following Putnam's operation often returned to a surprising degree, and some hope was offered that eventually the involuntary movements might be abolished without paralyzing the patient.

In the 1940s, Professor Russell Meyers pioneered operations aimed at islands of gray cells in the center of the brain. His principal target was a group of neurons called the globus pallidus. By means of a hazardous and daring operation, Meyers cut the nerves emerging from this structure, which was believed to modify the activity of the motor cortex itself. In other words, it was a secondary, or modulating, motor center rather than a primary one. Meyers' work gave great hope to the belief that the goal of relieving tremors and rigidity without paralyzing the patient would one day be achieved. Surgeons François Fenelon and Gérard Guiot in Paris confirmed and extended Meyers' primary efforts. However, practical progress was slow, and by the fall of 1951, when Joseph Cioppa of Philadelphia came to the University Hospital Clinic, seeking relief of his tremor, the immediate outlook appeared bleak. That year, Professor Roland MacKay, the editor of the *Yearbook of Neurology, Neurosurgery and Psychiatry* had stated that "Involuntary movements can be relieved only by substituting paralysis for the involuntary movement, and neurosurgery seems to have no application in this broad field."

The surgeon explained this to Cioppa, but also told him about an operation that had recently been developed by

Professor Earl Walker of the Johns Hopkins Medical School. He found that by cutting the motor pathway in the midbrain that is located halfway between the cerebral cortex and the spinal cord, the tremor could be lessened and total paralysis could be avoided, although some degree of weakness had to be expected. It was proposed to the patient that he undergo this operation. Cioppa said he would try anything—that he would rather be dead than continue to suffer the uncontrollable tremors.

On October 9, 1951, Joseph Cioppa was taken to an operating room in the University Hospital for a procedure that would never be completed, but one that would relieve his tremors and would be the first step in the history of the operation about to be performed on Janet.

The day that Cioppa was operated on, two young residents assisted the surgeon. One was Dr. Laurence Levy, who had come from England for neurosurgical training at New York University. The other resident was Dr. Aldo Morello, of Italy.[*]

A small opening the size of a half-dollar was made in the temporal portion of Cioppa's skull, just in front of the ear. The dura mater, the sac covering the brain, was opened and the temporal lobe was gently lifted so that the midbrain, which lies about two-and-one-half inches inside the skull, could be approached.

It was evident that the patient had previously had some kind of encephalitis, or brain infection, because the arachnoid, one of the protective coverings of the brain, was

[*] Dr. Levy is now Professor of Surgery at the University of Rhodesia, Union of South Africa. Dr. Morello is now Professor of Neurosurgery in Palermo, Sicily.

thickened and adhered to it, particularly in the region of the midbrain. It was necessary to open this thickened arachnoid with sharpened dissection. During this procedure a small artery inside of the arachnoid was cut, and it bled profusely. For several minutes the bleeding was so heavy, it appeared that the patient was in great danger. The surgeon turned to Dr. Morello, standing behind, and asked if he would go downstairs to the waiting family and tell them that the operation had taken a critical turn. Morello blanched, but said that he would go, and left the operating room.

Almost immediately, the surgeon was able to control the bleeding artery by squeezing it shut with a small silver clip. Once the bleeding was controlled, he went ahead with the dissection, visualizing the cerebral peduncle, preparing to cut the motor tracts in it.

However, it appeared that the tiny blood vessel he had been obliged to close off was the anterior choroidal artery. The function of this artery had been relatively unknown, but only recently the surgeon had read a long and detailed description of it in a medical journal. The article had reported the research of Dr. Leo Alexander of Boston, who pointed out that this tiny and seemingly esoteric blood vessel actually supplied blood to structures centrally placed in the brain that were related to modulation of motor activity. Therefore, the surgeon suggested to his assistant that the operation be terminated so that they could see what the effects of occluding this vessel were when the patient awoke from the anesthesia. Since Levy, although a resident, was the same age as the surgeon and a friend as well as an assistant, he urged him to be courageous and to go ahead and finish the operation he had started. However, the surgeon thought it was important to the patient to determine what the effects of closing off this blood vessel would be before proceeding with further surgery.

By the time this discussion was finished, Morello had returned from his distressing interview with the waiting family, and upon reentering the operating room, saw that the surgeon and his assistant were standing by the patient speaking and that there was no further hemorrhage from the wound, as there had been a few moments earlier when he left. He at once ejaculated, "My God! He's dead!" He was assured, however, that the patient was in good condition, and he concurred that it would be wise to observe the effects of the anterior choroidal artery occlusion, which it had been necessary to carry out, before cutting any additional motor pathways.

That evening, when the patient had recovered from his anesthesia and had fully regained consciousness, it was obvious that he was not shaking. It was a sleepless night for all, but the following morning, the surgeon and his assistants saw again that the patient was still free of his shaking, that he was not paralyzed, that he could speak, and that his intellect had not been damaged. The only change they could observe was the absence of the severe tremor that had been present previously.

That observation was the beginning of a very exciting time and of the further observations that led to the development of cryosurgery for dystonia and had brought Janet and the surgeon together on that day twenty years later.

In order to evaluate the possibility of employing purposeful occlusion of the anterior choroidal artery to relieve the tremor and the rigidity of Parkinsonism, months of research were necessary. With the cooperation of Professor Fred Mettler, whose basic research in this field had been carried out in the Department of Neurology at Columbia University College of Physicians and Surgeons, the surgeon was permitted to perform this operation on several baboons, the principal one being a five-hundred-pound animal named Rose. Dr. Mettler's meticulous examination of the baboons' brains after surgery strengthened the surgeon's hypothesis that occluding this artery damaged structures in the brain that contributed to tremor mechanisms in the human. These structures appeared to the surgeon to be crucial in alleviating tremor without producing paralysis in the patient.

Over the next few years, the surgeon performed this operation many times in human patients, and during one of these operations another important observation was made that contributed to the development of a surgical treatment for dystonia.

Donald Warren, a forty-two-year-old man who had been totally incapacitated by postencephalitic Parkinsonism since he was sixteen years old, was referred to the surgeon by Dr. Walter Freeman, who had been his professor of neurology in medical school, and whose exciting and rather flamboyant method of teaching had aroused his interest in neurology and in brain mechanisms. Warren's parents were approaching their seventies and had spent a quarter of a century devoting themselves to him from the time he became incapacitated. They were desperately seeking some way to lessen his incapacitation so that when they were no longer available to look after him, he would be able to help himself to some degree. The surgeon and the Warren family had many long talks, during which the risks and uncertainty of such a new procedure were explained. At that time, since the procedure was new, the exact statistics of each risk were still unknown. However, the surgeon explained that there would be at least a five percent risk of mortality, as well as a five percent risk of worsening of the patient's condition, or serious neurologic complication, adding to his already incapacitated state.

Since Donald was virtually speechless as a result of his longstanding infirmity, most of the conversation was with his parents. Finally the decision was made to operate on Donald.

In addition to his inability to walk, to rise from a chair, to feed himself, to hold a book, or to carry out any useful activity because of his severe tremor and the boardlike rigidity of his extremities, he had developed during the past fifteen years a marked, fixed deformity of his left hand. The hand was flexed at the wrist with his fingers painfully extended, and it was impossible to budge this hand even by the strongest maneuvers. Therefore, during the conversations before the operation, the surgeon mentioned to the parents that if the tremor and rigidity on the left side of the body were relieved by surgery, eventually some type of corrective orthopedic procedure might be done for this dystonic deformity of his left hand. This deformity was reminiscent of what he had observed in that neuromuscular disease of children, which he had been introduced to eight years before at Montefiore Hospital. Therefore, it seemed that the fixed deformity in the left hand of Donald Warren, which had been present for so many years, was obviously irreversible, and would require bone surgery and perhaps fusion at the wrist even to straighten it slightly.

Donald Warren underwent surgery September 29, 1953. By the following morning he was alert, could sit up in bed without difficulty, respond to questions, and revealed that the tremor and the rigidity of his left extremities had been totally relieved. Once again there was no sign of weakness or other difficulty with the left side. Within three days he could walk for the first time in more than ten years. He was discharged from the hospital two weeks later without any tremor or rigidity of the left side of the body. Moreover, much to the surgeon's surprise, there was some lessening of the deformity of his left hand, which appeared to be due to the loosening of some of the muscles that flexed the wrist. When the patient was seen two months after surgery, ambulatory and quite independent in his physical activities, the deformity of the left hand and wrist, which had been thought to be fixed and irreversible, had totally disappeared as a result of the relief of the rigidity of the musculature on that side of the body. The previously dystonic hand now had the loose, slender-fingered appearance of a lifelong pianist. Thus the surgeon learned that what he had thought to be a fixed deformity, involving muscles, tendons, joints, and bones, was really an abnormal posture without fixation and potentially reversible. This discovery of the result of anterior choroidal artery occlusion led him to conclude that the same type of deformities and abnormalities could be reversible in children who had dystonia musculorum deformans. Donald's operation led to the initiation of the investigation for the use of surgery in the globus pallidus and thalamus for dystonic movements and deformities and constituted another large step forward toward Janet's operation.

It seemed impossible at the time that by destroying a

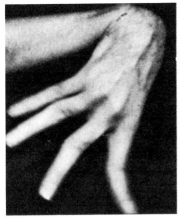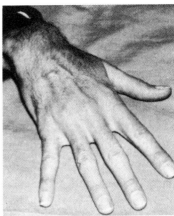

The previously dystonic hand, fixed in that abnormal position for sixteen years, now had the loose, slender-fingered appearance of a lifelong pianist.

small area several inches below the surface of the brain (parts of which had been damaged about three decades earlier by the encephalitic virus that scourged the world following World War I) torsions that had so long gripped Donald's hand could be stopped. And it also seemed impossible that this operation could be performed by a novice neurosurgeon, but it was true. Donald's tortured hand was unlocked, his dystonic posture totally reversed; and the key that unlocked it lay in an island of brain cells, neurons, closely guarded by being localized in the very center of the brain, an island known as the thalamus.

The word *thalamus* comes from the Greek *thálamos*, which means connubial couch. Whoever chose this name had the intuition of a great scientist, for the thalamus is a hotbed of sensorimotor activity. It is about the size of a walnut, although it is shaped like an egg. It consists of millions of nerve cells, each with hundreds of connections, and submits to thousands of nerve fibers passing through, going to and coming from virtually every other part of the brain. It serves as a data processor, or central communications area, interpreting sensory information that comes from muscles, skin, eyes, and ears. Sometimes this modulating, or controlling, apparatus of the thalamus is deranged. Oddly enough the derangement may be due not to a disease within the thalamus itself, but to a disease in other parts of the brain, which then sends staticlike messages or misinformation to the thalamus. When this happens, limbs may twist or shake or contort or bend or extend uncontrollably. Donald's hand provided the hint that surgery could cool the passion of the uncontrolled thalamus and still the tortured involuntary movements that it produced.

It was these two chance discoveries—the first in October of 1951, that tremor could be relieved totally without producing any paralysis, and the second in September of 1953, that a dystonic posture of longstanding could be totally reversed by the same type of brain surgery—that gave young Janet the hope of recovery on that May morning in 1971. Janet was the three hundred and twelfth dystonic child to lie in the quiet operating room, at once both fearful and brave, awaiting the surgeon whom she and her parents had decided to allow to probe her brain, to try, with her courageous assistance, to defuse the neuronal circuit that mysteriously locked her torso and limbs into painful, disabling contortions.

"Okay, Janet, we're ready to start now. You'll feel some pinpricks when we put the local anesthesia in your scalp. But it's only going to hurt for a few minutes. Hold tight, dear."

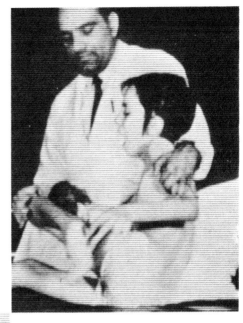

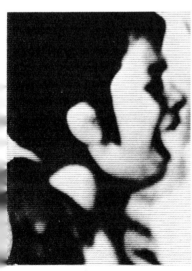

CHAPTER 2

A six-year-old child who has always been bright and active, raised in the brisk, hardy Western winters, and set free in the rolling gentle hills and farmlands in the summer, has little time or reason for morbid thoughts. She barely noticed during the fall of 1965 that when she ran her left foot twisted so that her toes pointed down and her ankle assumed the posture of an overextended ballet dancer's curvature. Even when her first grade teacher called her mother at home to report that Janet was limping, neither the teacher, nor Janet, nor her parents had any foreboding of the terror to come.

That barely noticeable twist of her foot was even then signaling an affliction that had been programmed into her brain and nervous system while she was still in her mother's womb. It had been programmed by a carrier of bad news in one of her ten thousand genes. That message, double helically encoded, delivered a message that would relentlessly predetermine future events, and the tragedy was set in motion.

It is paradoxical that the same gene, or one of its mates, almost invariably assures that the brain that will eventually send warped messages to convolute and twist muscles, will also be of superior intelligence. This adds irony and poignancy to the drama.

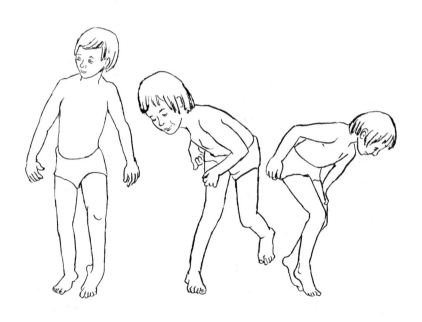

She barely noticed that when she ran, her left foot twisted.

Dystonia musculorum deformans is a specific, clinical syndrome that inflicts a combination of abnormal, uncontrollable involuntary movements and twisted, fixed postures of the arms and legs as well as of the neck and back (usually in small children between the ages of five and ten). These involuntary movements often become so severe, and the twisted, bizarre postures so grotesque, in an otherwise bright, alert, previously healthy child, as to cause great consternation, not only to the family but also to the physician called upon to explain the nature of this demon that has seemingly possessed the child.

The fact that most of its victims have a common genetic line was discovered in 1911 by Dr. H. Oppenheim, who found that a group of German children who had come under his care had several things in common. They had all developed normally until they reached an age between five and ten years. Then, although they were all intelligent, and no cause could be found, each had developed a twisted foot or a twisted hand, and gradually within the next year or two, had become incapacitated by twisting and torsion spasms of the entire body. Dr. Oppenheim noted that these German children all were descendents of Russian-Jewish immigrants who came from the southeastern part of Russia.

Some of the immigrants from that region settled in America, bringing with them the same genetic message, which has since been passed along to produce several generations of normal infants, who subsequently become racked and twisted after a few years of happy, healthy life. Only about half of the cases of dystonia musculorum deformans that have been recorded in the United States can be traced to a Russian site of origin. The other half appear to represent

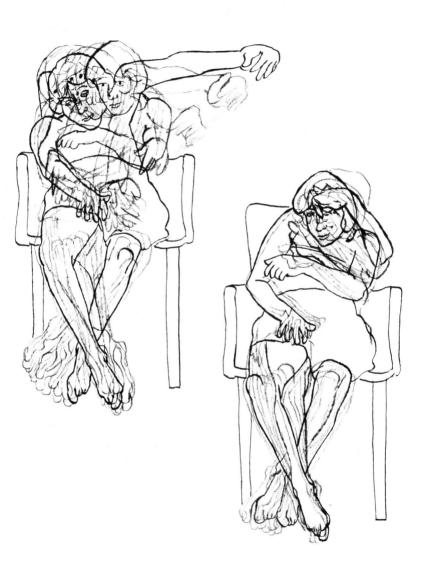

A thirty-six-year-old woman, totally incapacitated by abnormal postures and movements of far advanced dystonia.

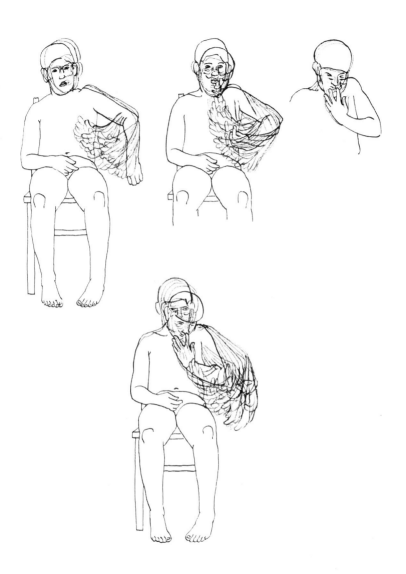

A nine-year-old boy, the son of the woman in the preceding picture, has noted the beginning symptoms of dystonia in his left arm.

genetic mutants, and are not confined to any particular ethnic group, but numbers WASPs, Puerto Ricans, and Blacks among the victims.

By the time Janet was carried in her mother's arms down the white, wooden steps of her modest home in Little Creek, Idaho, for the painful trip to the airport in Salt Lake City, she was already eleven years old. Until her first symptom appeared at age six, she had grown normally, and was active and bright, and weighed almost fifty pounds. When her mother carried her down the steps, five years later, in the spring of 1971, she weighed thirty-seven pounds, and her ribs stood out starkly under stretched parchment skin.

Although heavily sedated, she cried with pain. Her back arched, pushing her thin rib cage and stomach forward. Her left leg was doubled so that her left foot was stuck against her buttock, and could not be moved from that position because of the intense spasm of all the muscles of the leg and back. The right leg was stuck out like a ramrod, with the toes on the right foot twisted and curled under the sole of the foot. Her arms developed shaking and tremors if she tried to move them, and her face was an agonized mask. Janet had never been in an airplane before, but she was unable to express any interest in the large jet that she entered in Salt Lake City, and drugged, she dozed fitfully during the five-hour flight to Kennedy airport.

The following morning, Janet met the surgeon for the first time. She had already been examined by the assistant resident and the resident, but she screamed so with pain whenever one of them tried to move one of her twisted arms or legs, which resembled rigid, narrow branches of a small tree, that a detailed examination was not possible.

"Hi, Janet."

No reply.

"Hi, Janet. How about turning your face toward me so I can have a look at you?" She turned her face which was tear-stained, frightened, thin, with her expression somewhat dulled by the drugs she had been receiving for pain.

"Janet, I have to examine you a little bit today so that we can start trying to decide how we can help you."

"Don't touch me! Don't touch me! Don't touch my foot —I can't stand it!"

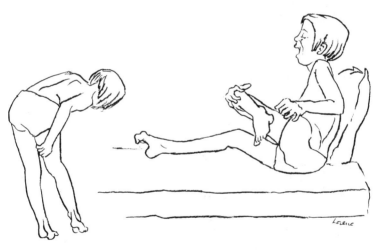

As the disease progressed, her back arched, and finally her left leg was doubled so that her left foot was stuck against her buttock. She could not be moved because of the intense spasm of all the muscles of her leg and back. Her right leg was stuck out like a ramrod, with her toes twisted and curled under the sole of her foot.

She screamed so with pain whenever one of the assistant surgeons tried to move one of her twisted arms or legs, that examination on that first day was impossible.

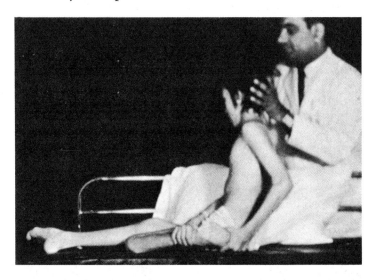

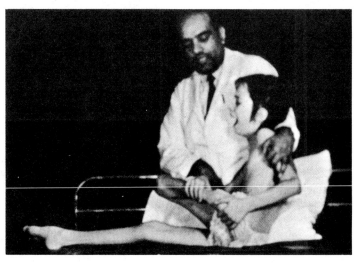

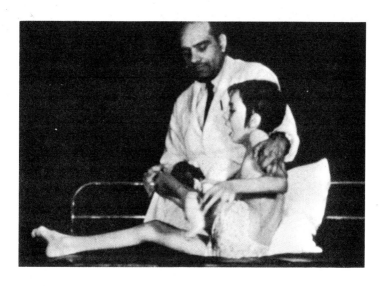

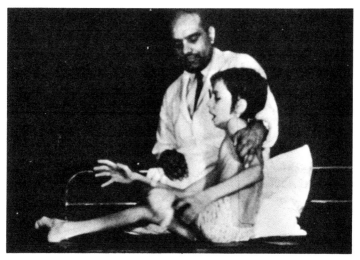

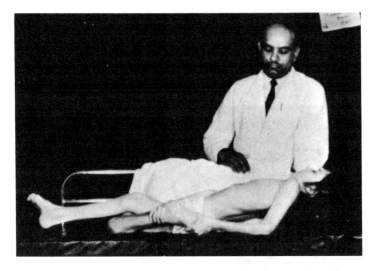

The resident had to return her to her grotesque, twisted position to await examination by the surgeon.

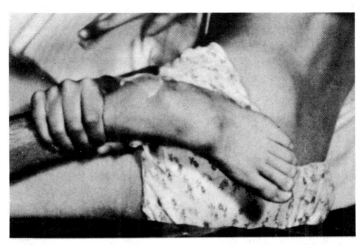

Left foot.

"I won't hurt you, Janet, I promise, but let me try to examine you so we can tell a little better what the situation is, and so that I can talk with you about what possibly might be done."

"NO! No! I don't want to be examined. Leave me alone!"

The surgeon gently placed his right hand under her shoulders and his left hand under her buttocks and tried to change her position from lying on her right side facing the wall to a supine position, with her lying on her back. Her screaming intensified, her back arched so much that the back of her head almost reached her buttocks; her pain was obviously agonizing.

"Try to relax, honey, and let us look at you—just a little." But any effort met the same resistance, making an attempt at examination

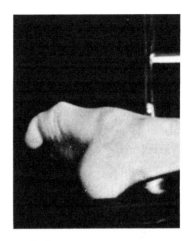

Right foot.

"NO! No! I don't want to be examined. Leave me alone!"

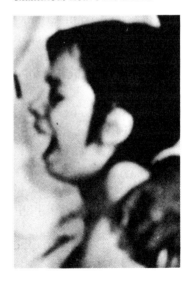

impossible. "Okay, Janet, we'll let you rest for a while and see you a little later."

After the surgeon left, others came. Attempts by the residents, the consulting neurologists, the clinical psychologist, and the surgeon to examine Janet later that day were all rebuffed. Actually, the surgeon already knew enough about Janet from the detailed history he had received from the referring physician, and by looking at her twisted body, to be relatively certain that her disease was dystonia. He knew that the tiny thirty-seven-pound body could not survive much longer unless some of the spasms that racked it were relieved. He knew, too, that Janet realized this as well and that by the following day she would be ready to be examined.

So, on that first day, the surgeon obtained more of Janet's story from her mother.

SURGEON: I want to talk to you a little bit about Janet. It's been impossible to examine her today, and we need to know more about her and how she reached this point. Janet is eleven years old. When she was born, was she perfectly normal?

JANET'S MOTHER: Perfectly normal. No problems.

SURGEON: Now, how old was she when you first noticed that something was wrong? Were you the first to notice?

JANET'S MOTHER: No, I wasn't. Janet was in first grade and her teacher called me at work and said Janet was limping. But Janet was not limping when she came home from school that day.

SURGEON: Did that happen on several occasions?

JANET'S MOTHER: Well, I didn't really notice her limping

at all and then three days later the teacher called me again, and I felt like she was going to turn me in for neglect or for being an unfit parent. She said, "You know, your daughter is limping. What are you going to do about this?" So then I came and got her at school and took her to the doctor.

SURGEON: On that day when you got her at school, you could see her limping?

JANET'S MOTHER: Yes. She had a slight limp on the left side and I took her to our G.P. He examined her quite thoroughly, and then he thought perhaps this might be the beginning of Legg-Calvé-Perthes [a hipbone disease]. So he sent her over to the hospital and he X-rayed her hips. But they were normal on the X-rays. So then we talked about Janet. Janet has always been kind of a hyperactive child, and he decided that this probably was just an emotional reaction—you know—first grade at school, and so forth. So he said to watch her for a few months and if her limping continued, I should bring her back in. He said sometimes Perthes disease does not always show up in X-rays. But from then on, she continued to limp. Her foot twisted when she walked. It got much worse—she started falling. And that's when we got real alarmed.

SURGEON: How much time did you wait before taking her back?

JANET'S MOTHER: Three months. We didn't take her right back when it got worse because he had said it was probably emotional, and we thought if we didn't pay a lot of attention to it . . .

SURGEON: So you didn't keep bugging Janet about it—you just kind of ignored it. Did Janet ever complain of it? Did she ever come to you and say, "There's something wrong with my leg. I'm limping"?

JANET'S MOTHER: I think she was somewhat concerned about it on occasions, but we just kind of ignored it. Then, when it became worse, we took her back to the doctor and he was worried because she was falling, and he immediately put her in the local hospital. And she had a complete physical—skull X-rays, spinal tap, all the blood work, and everything was negative. So then he came back to me and said, "I'm really worried because everything is negative." He sent her to a pediatrician because he was not a pediatrician—he was a general practitioner—and we went to the pediatrician and he examined her, and he in turn sent us to a psychiatrist. The psychiatrist looked at her for five minutes and asked, "How come this child hippityhops?" That made me mad, because this is all he did—five minutes, and he labeled her conversion hysteria on such a short evaluation—after he had talked to her, I'd say, for a few minutes in a room.

[Conversion hysteria is a psychiatric term used to describe a symptom which appears to be organic, but which has been caused by unconscious, unresolved psychologic conflicts that the patient is usually unaware of. For example, some cases of temporary blindness have been ascribed to a patient's fear of witnessing a situation that would be intolerable to him. Similarly, patients have been reported who appeared paralyzed—that is, unable to walk or to move their legs—who subsequently were found to be immobilized by unconscious fears, such as leaving the house or walking away from a protected environment. The name of the syndrome derives from the fact that these unconscious, unresolved conflicts or fears were converted into organic symptoms, such as blindness or paralysis. These symptoms are referred to by doctors as conversion hysteria or conversion reaction.]

And so we came back to our own doctor very unhappy with what the psychiatrist had said. He didn't recommend anything further be done. He just said that she was hysterical. Our doctor, our family doctor, wasn't satisfied with this, so he sent us to the hospital to a neurologist who was going to give her a neurological examination. And he examined her for about three hours. And he said he could find nothing wrong with her, and so he called down the doctor from Child Psychiatry. Then they decided that she needed hospitalization for psychiatric treatment. But they didn't have room for her, and so we took her home for a week or so. By this time she wasn't even able to walk; she was just lying in bed. That was the last time we ever saw Janet walking. Then the psychiatrist called after a week and said they could take her.

SURGEON: Now, up until that time did you mention the fact that you yourself had this tremor and deformity? Did you show your right hand to anybody?

JANET'S MOTHER: To everybody. I kept saying, "Is there a possibility that this means anything? You know, I've had this problem." Yes, I did.

SURGEON: So they all knew that you had a tremor and that when you tried to write, your hand twisted. Is that right?

JANET'S MOTHER: I didn't call it a tremor. Unless I extend my hand, the tremor doesn't come out. I told them I found it impossible to coordinate. But they never bothered to examine my hand or ask me anything about it. I kept saying, "You know, this may sound silly, but is there any possibility that there is a link between my problem with my hand and Janet's trouble?" And they all just kinda sloughed it off.

So anyway, she was admitted to the psychiatric ward for children and we were allowed to see her for the very most only one hour a week. And the first few weeks she was there weren't too bad. She adjusted pretty well. She seemed to be getting along. Emotionally, she accepted the place. But they weren't getting anywhere with her. So they were trying to think of all the different kinds of things—you know—what was wrong with her head. But they couldn't find anything wrong. And they just kept looking for things and they couldn't find anything.

SURGEON: Were you perfectly candid, frank with them all of the time?

JANET'S MOTHER: Right, right. In fact, I almost wish that we hadn't been. And we told them that we had had an episode—it was the only thing we could think of—about a year before, where a little boy in the neighborhood had been pulling the girls' pants down, and all of a sudden they had this big kick on, and said, "This is it." They started, you know, thinking it was probably a sex problem.

SURGEON: Now at this point, did they either tell you or Janet that? I mean, she had already been told it was hysteria. At what point did they start telling her that this was really some sexual problem? Did they actually tell her?

JANET'S MOTHER: I'll never forget it. They brought out all three of us—my husband, Janet, and myself—into the room. And they sat there and they started talking about

Janet taking her bath and playing with her brother. And all she did was sit there and cry, and I leaned over just to touch her with my hand and they told me to take my hand away. And they just kept on talking about what she knew about intercourse. And all she did was sob the whole time.

SURGEON: How old was Janet then?

JANET'S MOTHER: She was seven. And afterwards I got mad, and I said, "What right have you got to—you know— I'm her parent and I think I have the right to tell her about sex and the way I feel." They said I was a puritan and had puritan ideas on sex. All Janet did was sob. They sat there and accused her of playing with her brother in the bath-tub. I don't know what Janet told them when we weren't there. Janet added nothing to the conversation but tears. But they didn't really give us any suggestions. At that time they were experimenting with a behavior modification pro-gram of some sort. I wasn't ever quite clear as to all they were doing for her there because we were allowed such a short time visiting. We were never told of the exact course they were following. Then they told us that she was not ready to accept treatment and that it would take a good year to a year and a half to straighten her out. We said we couldn't afford it, you know, and they said they had funds available and they would take care of it.

Then, after she'd been there about four and a half months, they started in on this locking her in her room. But her symptoms just became progressively worse. Her left foot started to twist in—her right leg was not involved.

SURGEON: Was there an obvious progression of her neu-rologic symptoms while she was in the psychiatric ward?

JANET'S MOTHER: Mostly the internal twisting of her

foot. Finally we took her out of the hospital after that period in isolation. We did it against the wishes of the hospital. They were very angry with us.

SURGEON: Now, I want to get this straight. Did they tell you they were going to lock her in a room for a month? I mean, are you exaggerating? Literally locked in her room for a month?

JANET'S MOTHER: The door was not locked. But she was the only person in that room. There was a commode, but no radio, no TV set. It was a very small room—six by six— there was a bed and a commode—amen.

SURGEON: Any crayons or books or toys?

JANET'S MOTHER: In all honesty, I'm not sure.

SURGEON: Could you visit her during the month?

JANET'S MOTHER: One hour each Friday. All I remember is they told us—the door was not closed—they told us to tell her—and that they had told her also—that she could come out when she walked. And I remember after three weeks I went in, and I said, "Janet, this room is dirty"—they didn't dust—they wanted it to be dirty so she'd be sick of it—and I said, "How can you stand it?" You know, "Why don't you just get out, how can you stand it?" I was trying to encourage her, you know, to get up and walk, of course. And all she did was lie on the bed, and she said, "It's not so bad." She accepted it pretty well, just lying on the bed.

SURGEON: Did you ever ask her what she thought of the idea that she really could get better if she wanted to?

JANET'S MOTHER: We talked about it many times. I guess what I told her in essence was "God helps those who help themselves."

SURGEON: Did you think Janet's problem was psychological?

JANET'S MOTHER: At that time, yes. Because I thought we were at a teaching hospital. You know, who am I to know more than the professors. Yes, I guess I really did. I accepted their theory, but I didn't accept their methods.

SURGEON: Now, none of your other children by that time were showing any symptoms?

JANET'S MOTHER: No. That's been very recent.

SURGEON: How long ago was the hospitalization?

JANET'S MOTHER: That was five years ago.

SURGEON: Was she getting any psychotherapy? In other words, was anybody ironing out this sexual problem that she was supposed to have?

JANET'S MOTHER: In all honesty, I was not clued in to what they were doing. Janet told me that they put her up in front of TV cameras and that fifty doctors were staring at her, and that she had some type of shock treatment. And I believe this is correct.

SURGEON: Well, how did she happen to get out of this room? She couldn't walk . . .

JANET'S MOTHER: We got our doctor to call. We signed her out. We figured she'd had enough. We brought her home, and we did take their advice to this point: they said, "If you ever give her a walking aid, she'll never walk again." So she crawled to the school bus. She crawled into the classroom.

SURGEON: What kind of student was she?

JANET'S MOTHER: Good student—A's and B's.

SURGEON: But wasn't she in a psychiatric hospital again?

JANET'S MOTHER: Yes, she was admitted to a psychiatric ward at our local hospital last August, I believe it was, about the middle of August.

SURGEON: By that time, didn't you know she had dystonia?

JANET'S MOTHER: Well, one of the doctors we consulted said she might have dystonia, but he hadn't offered to do anything. That was the doctor who is the consultant for the crippled children's school where she went for three years. He told me he thought she might have dystonia. But he said all these diseases follow the same course, that there was no treatment for it—what's the difference, you've spent so much money now, what do you keep running to more doctors for? That was just a year ago last summer. A year and a half ago.

SURGEON: Okay. So how did you happen to get into the psychiatric unit at the hospital?

JANET'S MOTHER: A year ago June when school was out, she was becoming more and more spastic and more rigid. And I couldn't control her spasms and rigidity by drugs. One doctor I consulted said, "I don't know what to do. Don't even call me anymore. I just don't know." Then he said, "I want you to see another psychiatrist." And I said, "Don't give me another psychiatrist!" And he said, "Well, if you want me to help you, you've got to listen to me." And I said, "Ohhhh, we've had enough of psychiatrists." He said, "Well, this man also knows something about neurology." And by that time she was so bad, so spastic, so uncomfortable. We didn't know what else to do, so we went back to the local hospital, and they admitted her. She was as bad as she is now, with her left leg really curled up under her buttocks, but with more pain and more spastic.

One of the psychiatrists said, "I definitely think she has an organic disease." The other one who saw her—that was the one who had seen her the first time, five years ago, the one who talked about the hippity-hop, he was called in—and he said, "I still think she has a conversion reaction." And so they came up again with a diagnosis of conversion reaction. And they called in more psychologists. Then they started using hypnosis. And they explained to me that this was really very expensive and it was not to cure Janet in any way. It was to get her to relax her body. They had tried hypnosis five years ago, but she would not go under for them. This time, this particular psychologist gained Janet's confidence and she did—he hypnotized her. But she just kept getting worse.

SURGEON: Well, she really wouldn't let us examine her fully today, but there's no question in my mind that she has dystonia, and obviously the professor of neurology at the university finally came to that conclusion.

JANET'S MOTHER: Yes, a neurologist passing by in the hospital spotted what she had. There's no question in my mind. "A case right out of the book," he said.

SURGEON: That's right. She's right out of the book. Here you have the dystonic variant yourself and you have two children with neurologic symptoms. So we have to face the fact that it is dystonia and decide together what to do now. Let me tell you a little bit about dystonia and what we plan to do. As you know, since you've watched Janet, this is often a severely progressive disease. You've been lucky in that this slight dystonia that you have in your right hand is what we call a dystonic variant. That is, it's like a small piece of the disease that has affected your hand all these years, but hasn't really progressed and almost certainly never will, although there's no guarantee of that. But you do know that you passed along the gene that carries this abnormality and that Janet appears to have a virulent, almost malignant form of dystonia. It looks to us as though some of her joints, particularly her left knee and ankle, may even be already fixed by changes in the ligaments into those abnormal postures, and I'm not sure whether we can get them down or not. However, when we complete our examination, if we're still convinced that she has dystonia, then I'm going to suggest that we operate on her, so I want you to know a little bit about the surgery.

The operation that we perform is a brain operation. As you know, or probably heard, one-half of the brain controls the motor activity, the movements of the opposite side of the body, so that what we will do first is to operate on the right side of Janet's brain to try and relieve the muscle tension and rigidity on the left side of her body. If that is successful, it will cut down on the pain in her left arm and leg and make the muscles looser, and we might even be able to get that foot out from under her backside and eventually get her leg straight. However, that leg has become so severely deformed and has been in that position so long, I'd say there's only a fifty-fifty chance of getting it straight.

JANET'S MOTHER: When do you think you can operate on her, Doctor?

SURGEON: Well, today is Tuesday, and if we have any

success in examination tomorrow and there's no contra-indication, we'll try to go ahead by Thursday or Friday at the latest. But let me tell you about the possibilities of the surgery and the risks.

In any child whose symptoms are this far advanced and who already has fixed—what appear to be fixed—deformities, I would say there is about a fifty to sixty percent chance of being able to reverse the symptoms on the side of the body that we're operating for. If we're successful, then in a few months we could attempt to operate for the other side. However, you have to realize that each case is different. What we're going to do is put a tiny probe into the brain and destroy, by freezing, some islands of cells deep in the brain, which we've learned will often relieve this kind of muscle tension. Moreover, in order to try and determine how much has to be destroyed in each individual child, we must operate with the child awake, so that she can cooperate with us and let us examine her during surgery. This is going to be very difficult with Janet because of all she's been through, and because, in addition to being so upset, she's so physically weak and in constant pain. She's badly undernourished, but I don't think we can take the time to try and build her up. And besides, I doubt whether we could, unless we can first relieve some of these muscle spasms. One other thing that I have to tell you is that many times we've had to operate two or three times on one side of the body, and even then, of course, there's the chance that in this particular case we might not be successful.

JANET'S MOTHER: If there's a chance in a million, we have to take that chance.

SURGEON: Yes, I'm aware of that, but let me finish and tell you what the risks are. In addition to the risk that the operation won't be successful, there's a two percent chance of some complication that could lead to death, such as a stroke, for example. Statistically that's not a very big chance, but we have to consider it. Actually, since Janet's so sick, the risk of doing nothing in her particular case, I think, exceeds the risk of the operation. There's also an equal risk that surgical complications could cause paralysis on one side of her body, but in Janet's case that is not an overwhelming problem since she can't really use those extremities at the present time anyway. However, I want you to know that there are risks involved in brain surgery, and if she did have a stroke as a complication, then obviously any brain function could be affected—her speech or intelligence.

JANET'S MOTHER: What did you say the chances of that happening are?

SURGEON: Well, we've carried out this type of surgery in a little over seven thousand cases. Three hundred of those were kids with the same kind of problem that Janet has. The overall really serious risk is a little over two percent.

JANET'S MOTHER: I'd accept it if it were fifty percent and I know that Janet would too.

SURGEON: Okay, let me talk with her tomorrow and see if we can get a little further with our examination, and then I'll see you late tomorrow afternoon.

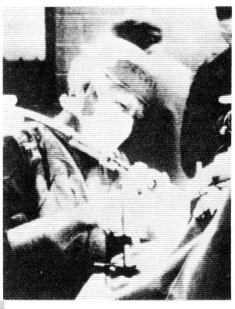

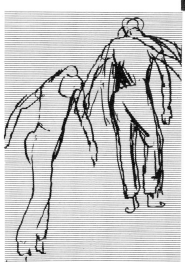

CHAPTER 3

It was like reliving a bad dream listening to Janet's story. A bright, normal kid, intelligent, highly motivated, active, becomes afflicted by peculiar, unexplainable symptoms. A limb twists—then relaxes—then twists again. Her back arches, she screams with pain, then it's gone—and her innocent laugh returns. Finally the limb remains twisted and the back contorted. No cause is apparent.

It's not that easy for a specialist to say he doesn't know why a child squirms as though she were bedeviled. It's even possible that that is the answer—that she's hysterical. She's now eleven and her twisted limb might be due to a twisted psyche.

Another patient of the surgeon's had gone that route, as had many of the dystonic kids who had preceded Janet. But David's case was one the surgeon could never forget.

David was referred for consideration of neurosurgical treatment when he was twenty-four, because of violent involuntary dystonic movements of his back, pelvis, and legs. He was neurologically normal until the age of seven when the toes of his right foot began to curl downward when he walked. Later the same year, involuntary bending of the right hand at the wrist with his fingers extending occurred when he attempted voluntary movements of the right hand.

47

By the age of ten his torso had become involved and he had involuntary, jerky, jumping movements of the left hip. These increased to involve the entire pelvis, so that during walking, the pelvis was constantly thrust backward and forward. Between the ages of seven and twenty-two, this young man was examined in major pediatric clinics. Because of the bizarre nature of his symptoms, particularly the involuntary movements of the pelvis, the diagnosis remained questionable as to whether his problems were physiological or psychological in origin.

During the crucial phase of adolescence and young manhood, he was told by several doctors that his symptoms were hysterical and was provided with various explanations of his behavior. It would be unusual if the psychiatric testing in this type of patient did not reveal neurotic traits, anxieties, and other evidences of emotional disturbances. The presence in the home of a distorted, writhing child, who is racked by involuntary movements that neither he nor his parents understand, invariably leads to frustration, hostility, and feelings of guilt on both sides. The infliction of a diagnosis of hysteria in this type of case and an attempt to ascribe the symptoms to family relationships augment the frustration and anguish of the patient and those around him.

By the age of seventeen, David was totally incapacitated. At that time a diagnosis of psychoneurosis, conversion hysteria, was made and he was admitted to a psychiatric hospital for treatment. Dystonia is often a bizarre and an unpredictable disease. In its early stages the involuntary movements come and go. Usually the abnormal postures,

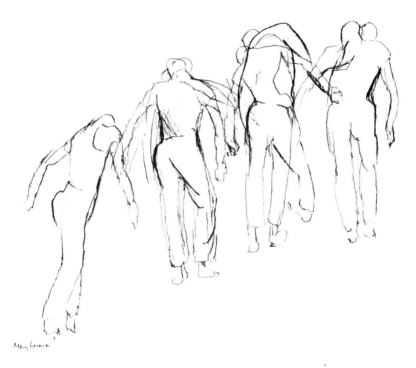

Mary Lorence

Twenty-two-year-old David, in whom dystonia twisted his back, produced involuntary movements of his pelvis, and incapacitated him physically and socially.

which are due to simultaneous contractions of antagonistic muscles—contractions of flexors and extensors at the same time—does not appear until the patient stands or attempts voluntary movement. When the patient is calm, sitting in a chair, the movements are not obvious. As with all involuntary movements, including the tremor of Parkinsonism, the involuntary movements are usually worse when the patient is tense or under emotional duress. Consequently, in the early stages of the disease, it may be very difficult to diagnose. Moreover, because of the tendency of symptoms to come and go and to become worse when a patient is excited, and because the patient remains intellectually normal, there is often an inclination to believe that the origin of the symptoms may be psychological, that is, due to deep, unexpressed emotional problems.

In some persons who have emotional difficulties that are not expressed verbally, bodily symptoms may appear that are psychiatric or hysterical in origin. For example, a patient who may be fearful about going outdoors for some obscure emotional reason may develop an inability to use his legs. This is called a conversion of unstated psychological problems into physical symptoms and accounts for the name of conversion hysteria.

So David was admitted to a psychiatric hospital and was seen three times a week in psychotherapeutic interviews, which amounted to one hundred forty-six therapeutic psychiatric sessions. The psychiatric interpretation of his illness was based on the doctor's opinion that his symptoms had an exhibitionistic quality—that his manner of walking caused people to look at him. The following is the statement made by David's psychiatrist at the time of his discharge from the mental hospital:

DAVID

When this seventeen-year-old single, white male was admitted, he had a severe motor disturbance in walking, giving him a grotesque, uncoordinated gait so that his arms and legs and trunk seemed to have no control. They would flail about, his trunk would move backwards and forwards so that his buttocks would be protruding or his pelvic area protruding in front, and this would alternate back and forth. His head was always bent forward so that he was looking down toward the ground. Yet, when he was sitting or lying down, he would be apparently without symptoms. His right hand, when in use, would be flexed at the wrist and his hand would be formed in a fist. This difficulty had been present since the patient was nine years old, and has gradually progressed in severity.

The patient was seen in psychotherapeutic interviews three times a week; the interviews being a half hour in duration. In all, he had 146 therapeutic sessions while at the hospital. During this time, a good deal of historical data was obtained, which is elsewhere in the record. He soon got into his feelings of hostility toward his father, especially, as well as his mother and sister. He complained bitterly about their mistreating him. In time, he began to see his own provocative behavior inviting punishment. It was later in his treatment that he related to his own masochistic drives and he could see how scratching his own skin at times was related to this. He gained insight into the exhibitionistic quality of his symptoms and talked a good deal about how he wanted everyone to notice him, to look up to him, to think of him as a great man. He felt his way of

51

walking was forcing people to look at him. This exhibitionism, at no time during his stay in the hospital, was related, in his thinking, to his fear of touching his own penis.

The difficulties with his right hand meant that he could never masturbate with his right hand. In masturbation, he would use his left hand or, more commonly, masturbate on the pillow. Whenever he touched his penis with his right hand, he lost his sexual desire. This was obviously related to his castration anxiety and he was behaving as though he was castrated and had no penis.

He learned in good time a good deal about the meaning of his symptoms, how his sticking his stomach out was, on the one hand, imitating his mother's pregnancy with his younger sister, whereas, on the other hand, it was putting his penis forward and asserting himself as a man. Inevitably, whenever he sticks his stomach out, he withdraws it rapidly and sticks his buttocks out. He could see in time how this was, in part, related to his fear that harm would be done to his penis, when it is stuck out, and sticking out his anus prominently was an invitation for sexual attack from the rear. This would protect his penis. In his associations, it was clearly related to his own habit of offering his mother and grandmother his anus to wash, so that they wouldn't wash his penis.

He gained a good deal of insight into his feminine identification and his attraction to men. His forward movement of the penis tells us that it also had the purpose of closing off his anus from attack from the rear.

He thought of himself in grandiose terms, as a great person, powerful, who could do things no one else could do. He felt by his walk that he forced people to do things for him, such as drive him places, look at him, etc. At no time could he accept the weakness involved. He also gained a good deal of insight into the defensive nature of his symptoms, hiding especially his hostile and aggressive thoughts and feelings.

During his stay, he recalled many memories which obviously were related to sexual thoughts about his mother from childhood but these were not pulled together and he never fully accepted his sexual wish toward his mother, while he was in the hospital.

Although the patient's gait didn't improve during his stay, his relationship with his family was much better, so that he was more comfortable being with his parents and sister at the time he left the hospital. *It seems he wasn't at all ready to give up his symptoms as yet because they were giving him much too much gratification to be relinquished.* [Italics the author's.] This would be the area that had to be worked on a great deal in his future treatment.

DIAGNOSIS ON DISCHARGE: psychoneurosis, conversion hysteria
CONDITION ON DISCHARGE: improved

After his discharge from psychiatric therapy, David's symptoms continued to progress and he became totally disabled. He was unable to carry out ordinary daily activities of self-care, and for two years prior to referral to the surgeon, he received rehabilitation and occupational therapy. During that time, a neurologic consultant in one of the rehabilitation centers told David that he suffered from dystonia. He was sent to several of the major neurologic clinics in New York and the diagnosis was confirmed.

Highly motivated, as are all of these kids, he went to work for Abilities, Inc., located in Albertson, Long Island. While working in their factory, which employs only disabled people, he came to the attention of the director, Mr. Henry Viscardi, Jr., as well as Dr. Howard Rusk, Director of the Institute of Rehabilitation of New York University. They referred him to the surgeon for evaluation for possible surgery in an attempt to alleviate his far-advanced dystonic symptoms. By the time David was seen by the surgeon and his service, he was not only totally incapacitated, but also confused about the conflicting medical and psychiatric opinions that he had received between ages seven and twenty-four. He was bitter, hostile, and totally distrustful of virtually all doctors.

When he was first seen by the surgeon in 1958, the fact that he had dystonia was readily apparent. However, although the possibility of surgical therapy was discussed, the surgeon believed that David had already undergone too many frustrations and disappointments to be able to withstand the disillusionment that might follow if he were operated on and his symptoms were not alleviated. For this reason, he was advised to think things over for a few months—to consider the fact that the operation had about a sixty percent chance of relieving his symptoms and that at least two operations would be required, one for each side of his body. He was also told that there would be a risk to his life of about two percent each time he was operated on, and, finally, that he would have to face the fact that he might undergo two or more operations without achieving the type of relief he required.

During the next few months, David consulted with Dr. Rusk and Mr. Viscardi several times. He went to other clinics and every major medical center in New York City to have the diagnosis confirmed. Finally, in early 1959, he entered the hospital for surgery.

The first operation was performed on the right side of his brain in order to relieve the symptoms on the left side of his body. It appeared to be immediately successful, with abolition of the involuntary movements on the left side and without any postoperative difficulties. However, within two weeks, all of the symptoms had returned, and with them came much of the despair and disillusionment that had been feared. However, David agreed to one more try, and two weeks after the first operation, a second was performed, again on the right side of the brain, enlarging the lesion or tissue destruction, in the right thalamus. This time the symptoms in his left extremities disappeared and did not recur. Three months later, a similar procedure was carried out on the left side of the brain, again successfully.

From that time to this, the thirteenth anniversary of these operations, David has remained essentially normal. He was able to leave Abilities, Inc. and resume a physically normal life. The following is a letter from Mr. Viscardi:

December 29, 1962

My dear Doctor,

I thought it would please you to know that last week David shipped out as a crew member of the *Santa Sylvia* of the Grace Lines. He is now in the Caribbean and not expected back for a month.

It has been a long-cherished ambition of his to go to sea, and now, because of you and those who have believed in him, this almost impossible goal has been realized. Add it to the little Christmas presents under your tree . . .

Today, in 1972, David is thirty-nine. He has a somewhat gangly, loose appearance when he walks, but does not demonstrate any neurologic abnormality. In recent years he has worked at an airport, where he drives a heavy truck. He remains fully independent not only in activities of daily living, but in his work, which requires great physical effort and mental concentration. When would David, now normal, forget his writhing, lonely, haunted childhood years? When would he forget the tortured, misused, unending analysis of his childish sexual fantasies? When would he awake without the fear that today, this day, his foot might twist again? When? Never, that's when.

It is often true that when such patients have been restored to physical normalcy, they require continued support, guidance, and encouragement to reenter a world from which they have been isolated by their disease for many, many years. One of the most difficult things persons with involuntary movement disorders have to contend with is social alienation. Centuries ago, many such people were burned at the stake as witches, because it was thought that their grotesque behavior was due to possession of their bodies by demons. There was no evidence that they were possessed, but the sight of these disfigured, tortured beings was often more than their neighbors could bear. Although things have changed a great deal since then, people with visible symptoms still become isolated, and are made to feel animalesque and despised. In cases in which they have been led to believe that their symptoms are due to emotional factors, they bear great guilt because they are unable to control them. Finally, people who have been fortunate enough to be relieved of their torsion and spasms and contorted limbs are often left with an image of themselves in their prior, alienated state. Some, then, require psychiatric counseling and help, and benefit from it.

Neurosurgical therapy and psychiatric therapy carry great risks as well as possibilities for benefit. Neither should be resorted to unless there is absolute indication that a condition exists to which the possibility of benefit outweighs the risks. When adequate medical therapy becomes available for dystonia, as it has for Parkinsonism, there will be no need for any patient to assume the risks of brain surgery. Moreover, until a positive diagnosis was established, David would have been better off without therapy of any kind—psychiatric or neurosurgic. Such an approach is a last resort, but it was one that Janet—eleven years old, a thirty-seven-pound frail, twisted, frightened child—now faced.

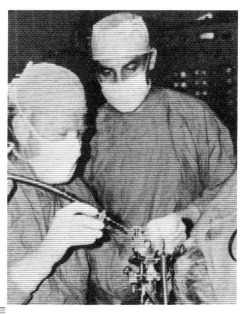

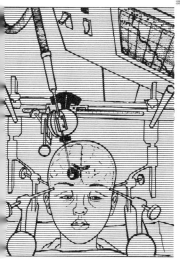

CHAPTER 4

Wednesday morning. The morning rounds were just about over, and a group stood in the corridor of the third floor of Kane Pavilion outside of Room 356. "I think it's best that I speak with Janet alone this morning." The associate surgeons, residents, nurses, speech therapists, physical therapists, and two visiting surgeons turned to go to their own tasks.

In Room 356 lay Janet, still tearful. Her mother, sitting by her bedside constantly holding the painful left foot, which is pressed against Janet's buttock, from time to time strokes her gently. In the other bed of Room 356 lay Susan, at fourteen a veteran in the battle against dystonia. Originally completely disabled by the disease, she has already been operated on three times. The ventral lateral nucleus of the thalamus on the right side of the brain was operated on first, then the same area on the left. Being incompletely relieved, six months later a more posterior portion of the thalamus on the left side of the brain was operated on, and the right extremities now appear normal. Her left arm, however, was still bent upwards and was twisted so that the elbow crossed the chest and her left fist was plastered against the outer portion of her left shoulder. She, too, occasionally cried with pain. But she was now hopeful and cheerful and greeted the surgeon as he came through the door.

"Morning, Doctor. When do we go again?" she called. Susan's parents were standing at the foot of the bed, tense but also hopeful.

"Tomorrow morning, Susan. We'll start about nine o'clock. I hope that number four will be the last and that we'll get that arm down and send you back to school."

"I'm sure it will be okay, Doctor. Thanks a lot."

The surgeon indicated to Susan's parents that he'd like to chat with them in his office after he'd had a chance to speak to Susan's roommate, Janet, alone. Janet's mother gradually loosened her gentle grip on Janet's contorted foot, stood, and at a nod from the surgeon, followed Susan's parents out to the hall.

"Good morning, Janet." Janet turned her face to the wall with no reply. "Good morning, honey. How did you sleep last night?"

"I didn't sleep. I hurt too much."

"How about turning your face toward me, sweetheart, so we can talk to each other?"

"No."

The surgeon drew a chair next to the bed, placing it at the head of the bed in order to look at Janet's face. "Janet, you've come a long way to try to get some help. The reason that we're here is to try and do just that. But the type of problem you have is different from most illnesses. At least at the present time, we need your help very much if we're going to make any progress. The type of surgery we're going to talk about requires your cooperation, or we can't do it. So since you've had so much trouble and you hurt so much, and you've come such a long way, it's just a little bit more to turn around so that you and I can get to the reason that you're here and try to do something about it." By this time, although she was still facing the wall, Janet had begun quietly to cry. "Well, Janet, how about it?"

"No. I don't want to talk. I've heard that stuff before about having to help myself. I can't help myself, and I don't want to talk about it."

"I'm only talking about your cooperation with us, Janet. You knew very well when you came here you thought an operation might help you. The doctor at home explained that to you before you came, and you made that decision to come. When I speak about your help, I mean first of all, your understanding of your own situation, and what we might be able to do for you. But we can't do anything unless you first understand what we plan to do, and want it done, and are willing to go ahead with it."

"No. I'm sorry I came. Just leave me alone."

"Janet, I know you've been through a lot. I know that you're a sick little girl, that you've had a lot of pain, and that you've had a tough time. There's nobody in the whole world that wants to help you more than I do. But I can only ask you to turn around and talk to me so that we can get ahead with our goal. If you won't talk to me, then you might as well go home."

"You're right—I want to go home. I don't want to talk to you. I just want to be left alone."

"Okay, Janet, if you're so goddamn smart, go back to Idaho." The surgeon rose, put the chair back into place and walked out.

In the corridor outside the room, alone, anxious, as frightened as Janet, stood her mother. "Well, Doctor, what did she say?"

"I really couldn't get her to talk to me. She's upset and frightened and confused and very bitter about everything. I don't think I can be totally permissive with her, for if we make the decision to go ahead, I'll have to be able to control her totally when we're in the operating room, or she won't be able to go through the procedure awake and cooperate with us. For a little while, I'll have to be a bit tough with her so that she understands and has some faith that we are trying to do everything we can and that there's some chance for her to get better. I'm sure that she'll come around. Lots of kids have begun like this, but their depth of understanding ultimately is unbelievable. However, she's got to make the decision, and she can't do that until she understands more about the situation. I'm sure she'll think about it, and I'll get a chance to talk to her again. In the meantime, you'll just have to be patient."

"I've waited a long time, Doctor, I can be patient."

"Okay, then we'll probably be seeing each other later in the day."

What does a bright, frightened, eleven-year-old child think when she's helpless, totally ill, deformed, and incapacitated for four of her eleven years? What does she think when she wants to turn away and can't? What does she think when she wants to use her contorted legs and arms that are facing the other way, and she's powerless to use them? What does she think when she knows that she's two thousand miles from home and that the only hope that's offered to her is brain surgery?

Anyone knows that having your brain operated on must

be a hell of a thing to go through. Just the indignity of a shaved head is enough to make one shudder. The physical reality of an opening in your skull is not an easy, pleasant fact to grasp. But most of all, the brain was put in that hard case so that it would remain inviolate, with all its memories and secrets, thoughts and ideas, with its personality and identity locked away, in the interaction of its millions of neurons. It's not an easy decision to make, to allow someone to operate on your brain. Being eleven years old, and having been persuaded that your limbs twisted because you wanted attention and had some sexual obsession at age seven and that you were hysterical, doesn't make it any easier. What was Janet thinking, lying there in that bed? She was thinking that she's desperate and that she wants to get well, and that she'll take any chance and do anything to try to help herself. And later that afternoon, she sent for the surgeon to tell him so.

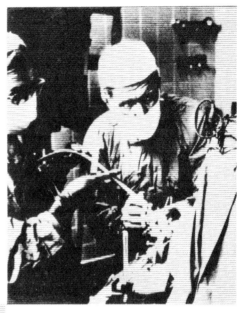

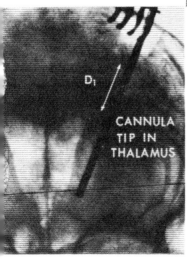

D₁

CANNULA
TIP IN
THALAMUS

CHAPTER 5

How does one decide to place for the first time an instrument deep in a child's brain and destroy part of it? It's not just a question of overcoming the technical difficulties, which can always be worked out in the laboratory. It's a more profound, moral question than that, because only human beings have this disease. Monkeys or cats or rabbits or guinea pigs don't have dystonia. So far, scientists have not been able to produce it in these animals experimentally. So the rationale for operating on the brain of a dystonic child, no matter how well founded on empiricism, or experience, could not first be put to the test in animals.

If it were ever to be done for the first time, it had to be done on a human victim of the disease.

How does one decide to risk that first time in a child? The first child with dystonia musculorum deformans he had operated on was also an eleven-year-old girl. Her disease started when she was eight and progressed rapidly so that by the time she was ten she was totally helpless. Her symptoms were somewhat unique in that, in addition to the abnormal postures, all four limbs and her head and neck were constantly, violently, thrown by involuntary movements. These went on night and day until she slept from utter exhaustion or was put to sleep with a modified anesthetic medication.

Her family doctor had suggested every medication and physical therapy that he thought might help. But her violent movements and spasms progressed relentlessly. Then, having read in a medical journal of the surgeon's hopeful results from a new approach to involuntary movement disorders, he called the surgeon and asked him to see the child. He believed the patient's condition was desperate and urged the consideration of some heroic measure, if there seemed to be any chance for success.

When he first saw this child and spoke to her parents, he told them that he thought there was a slight possibility of stopping these horrible movements, which could not otherwise be controlled, by the type of brain surgery he had developed for Parkinsonism. However, he pleaded for more time, and admitted that in a child, he could not yet clearly delineate the risks. He also admitted that he really did not know how to decide to make this first trial in their child.

Within a week her parents were back. They had decided, and they were there to tell him of their decision.

"Either you make the effort and try to relieve our daughter by this brain operation, or we're going home and turn on the gas. We mean it—the whole family. We can't stand it any longer."

Even now, fifteen years later, he believed they would have done just that. They'd watched their child suffer as long as they could bear it. He could understand why they were at the point of turning on the gas.

There was a reasonable scientific rationale back then, in 1956, for him to believe that by destroying a part of the thalamus her symptoms might be relieved. Therefore, the main problem was not the physiological basis of the surgical approach, but rather the larger moral question. Does one have the right to do this for the first time? Who has the right to decide? His criterion for making that decision centered on the individual, the child who had dystonia. His ultimate concern was with her welfare. All of his training, study, preparation had no other meaning, at that moment, other than to help that particular child. Did the operation offer her a chance for less pain, for less suffering, a possibility of rehabilitation that could not be found elsewhere? The procedure could not be carried out in an attempt to gain information that might help future children, or in an attempt to learn more about the human brain, or in an attempt to learn more about dystonia. If there were secondary gains, so much the better. But the only possible reason for performing that first operation was to alleviate the child's suffering.

Fifteen years later, having just left Janet, his concern was still the same. Could the operation reasonably be expected to help this child? Was he entitled to let this child take the risk? Which risk was greater, the disease or brain surgery? He knew the answer to these questions now, but the anxiety that accompanied the responsibility of the decision was reborn each time. He used to wonder when that anxiety, tension, and pain of decision involving the ultimate value, a single life, would disappear.

He knew the answer to that question now. When? Never.

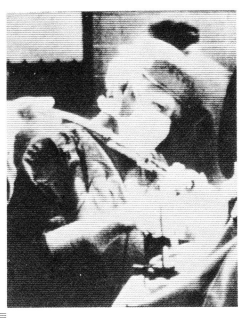

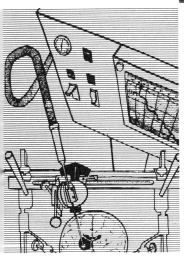

CHAPTER 6

Susan's parents were seated in the surgeon's office, which was two floors beneath the room where Janet and Susan lay in adjacent beds. While the surgeon and her parents chatted below, Susan, the fourteen-year-old veteran of eight years of dystonia and three brain operations, was comforting and counseling eleven-year-old Janet—and probably giving her more considered, mature, intelligent insight into her problem than anyone else had yet been able to give.

The surgeon pulled his chair around to the front of his desk, so that the desk did not come between the couple and himself.

SURGEON: Well, here we are again. I'm certain that by now you know as much about the situation as I do, but I am anxious to discuss Susan's operation tomorrow. That is, should we really go ahead—or settle for the improvement she's gotten so far?

They both spontaneously objected. Susan's father even got up from his chair.

SUSAN'S FATHER: Oh, for God's sake, don't say that! We're all ready for the operation, and Susan would be fantastically disappointed. She couldn't wait to get here this time.

SURGEON: Yes, I know that—and I don't say we shouldn't go ahead. All I want to do is to re-discuss the situation and make certain you, and Susan, too, understand the fact that we're at the point where she doesn't have to take the risk. She's not entirely well, but she's so much better that even though we all feel she should go ahead tomorrow, I don't think we should do so without going over the situation once more.

SUSAN'S FATHER: Okay, Doctor, we'll re-discuss it if you want to, but we're anxious to go ahead. Odd, to tell you the truth, since we've already made up our minds about Susan, we've been more concerned the past day about Janet and her mother.

SURGEON: Yes, I guess everybody around the place is really distressed about Janet at the moment. She's such a pitiful little thing, and in such pain that everyone's upset and concerned about her.

SUSAN'S MOTHER: The fantastic thing about Janet's mother is that she's able to go through this alone.

SURGEON: Well, she really isn't alone. Her own mother is here with her, and since they need help, we've gotten a local convent to put them up. So I think she's getting as much support—morally and every other way—as is possible.

SUSAN'S MOTHER: Oh, I know that, but I would think it would be so tough without her husband here. You know, she's gone through exactly the same suffering that we have, but had to do a lot of it by herself. We've been fortunate enough to be able to take the time and be here together.

SURGEON: Yes, you're a lot luckier than most in that regard.

SUSAN'S FATHER: The thing that makes me so goddamn

mad is the fact that Janet and Susan, and we, us too, have been put through the ringer by the medical profession before we ever got here, and the stories are so alike, you'd almost think it had come off the same Xerox machine.

SURGEON: Well, I'm not sure the whole medical profession has put you through the ringer. But what do you mean that your stories are so much alike?

SUSAN'S MOTHER: Well, mainly, I guess, it's the psychiatric bit. The fact that these kids were told their problems were hysterical for such a long time and that nobody really seemed to be interested in tracking the problem down.

SUSAN'S FATHER: It's the complacency—not the ignorance. You go to so many doors, and all the doors are open but only a quarter open. The first trouble was not believing she was physically ill, and for a couple of years, putting her—and us—through the psychological business. And then, after discovering what she had, after the diagnosis was made, they still won't believe it. It's the vanity of these physicians who really have great power—particularly the chiefs and professors, that's so hard to take. Many of them really seem more interested in demonstrating their own erudition and cleverness than in dealing with the problem of the patient.

SURGEON: When you say "they," who do you mean?

SUSAN'S FATHER: The pediatrician, the neurologist, the psychologists who saw her—they wouldn't believe she had dystonia.

SURGEON: Well, somebody must believe it. Who diagnosed it?

SUSAN'S MOTHER: I don't blame them for not recognizing it, originally I mean, because of what we've been through.

I just don't want any doctor to go away with the thought that our child developed certain symptoms and that we took her to a doctor, and he said, "Your child has dystonia." And that that was the beginning of the story. I don't want any doctor to think that. I want them to know about the years—not the visits, not the days, not the weeks, but the years—that led to our getting here to your office. Even when the diagnosis was finally made, we were simply told it's hopeless, there's nothing to be done. We once read in the paper an article about a report you delivered to the American Medical Association. It described your development of cryosurgery for certain brain operations and even showed pictures of some children and adults you had operated on. When we asked the neurologist, he said, "Oh, I don't believe in surgery for this sort of thing." That's what I mean by vanity of power! Why couldn't he have said, "Well, that type of surgery doesn't always work" or "It has too much risk in my opinion." But to say he just doesn't believe in it seems ridiculous. Why couldn't he be more humane? We're intelligent. It's our problem. Why couldn't they at least give us the facts and let us share in the decision. It's the arrogance—the arrogance of power that makes us bitter. This is what disturbs me—and Janet's mother has gone through exactly the same thing.

SURGEON: Okay. Then you tell me about it. Tell me what happened first, and then each incident that followed. I want to know exactly in chronological order the development of Susan's symptoms.

SUSAN'S MOTHER: In October of 1968 Susan developed a limp. I immediately took her to the pediatrician, which is a mother's first thought . . .

SURGEON: And this is in Dallas?

SUSAN'S MOTHER: Right. In Dallas—a suburb of Dallas. She was close to being eleven. He examined her, gave her a general physical exam, and said he didn't see anything wrong, but I should take her to a neurologist because there was something wrong with her balance. I took her to a neurologist . . .

SURGEON: Did he pick the neurologist? I mean, he was a man that you knew was qualified?

SUSAN'S MOTHER: Yes.

SUSAN'S FATHER: He happened to be the chief neurologist at the big hospital there.

SUSAN'S MOTHER: And he had a private practice in our area. He examined her and he said he could find nothing wrong with her physically, that it might be just a nervous type of thing or something like that. He gave me some medication, which I assume, well, which I know, was a muscle relaxer, a tranquilizer. It didn't go away, it got worse. I took her back to the pediatrician. He said that there was nothing wrong with her. I'm trying to condense the best I can. The symptoms kept appearing.

SURGEON: What were the symptoms?

SUSAN'S MOTHER: Tremor started . . . in her hand . . . her arms . . .

SURGEON: Where? It was still on her left side at that time?

SUSAN'S MOTHER: I believe so. Her neck started turning . . . The whole progression of symptoms started in.

SURGEON: So, how far along were you—what month were you in?

SUSAN'S MOTHER: Well, I would say October. By the end

79

of November, the doctor told me he thought it was an emotional problem.

SURGEON: But was her neck turning by that time?

SUSAN'S MOTHER: No, it was not.

SUSAN'S FATHER: No, her foot. She began with her foot.

SURGEON: And was her foot turning in?

SUSAN'S MOTHER: Yes, right. It started to turn in, but it was more of the arched foot. She started to limp. He felt there was nothing physically wrong with her. The neurologist felt there was nothing physically wrong. But I kept . . .

SURGEON: What was the nature of the emotional problem as he saw it?

SUSAN'S MOTHER: Well, he said—we went to this psychologist.

SUSAN'S FATHER: Let me clarify this. He was part of a group clinic, so he had a psychiatrist, a neurologist, a pediatric neurologist there. He had ample resources—like you and your staff.

SUSAN'S MOTHER: He talked to Susan. He asked, you know, about our family.

SURGEON: How old was Susan at the time?

SUSAN'S MOTHER: Going on eleven. It was November. No, she was ten. This was the end of November and she was eleven the following January. He looked at Susan and observed her and he started asking questions about the family. He went back into our family history. He said my husband would have to come there, which he agreed to do. He went into, for instance, that Fred was born in Germany. His father was in a concentration camp. He had a hard time getting out of Germany during the war. All these things connected with our family. I said he was a very strict father. The children were disciplined at home, et cetera. The usual things that you talk about. And then Fred came in to see him, too. He said we all needed psychological testing. He said Susan was doing this to get attention.

SURGEON: Now at this point were you prepared to accept the fact that this was emotional?

SUSAN'S FATHER: I was prepared. I was prepared to accept any . . .

SURGEON: I mean, had Susan had problems?

SUSAN'S MOTHER: No, Susan hadn't had an emotional problem in her life. I think she was the most well-adjusted, sweetest child I ever met. She was no problem at school. There was no problem . . .

SUSAN'S FATHER: She was getting all A's at school, she was president of her class, she was a leader among her friends.

SUSAN'S MOTHER: We have a boy who is now six years old—eight years younger than Susan. When the doctor said she was doing this for attention, we thought maybe there was some conflict because after eight years there was a baby in the house, and maybe that had some effect on her —being the eldest child.

SURGEON: Okay. But you personally had not been aware of any emotional problem?

SUSAN'S MOTHER: I didn't see any emotional problem . . .

SURGEON: On the other hand, an authority told you, and you accepted it.

SUSAN'S MOTHER: Right. Many authorities told me. The psychologist said Susan was doing it for attention, and the way to treat it was not to reinforce her behavior by acknowledging what she was doing. In other words, don't pay attention to her, and it will go away. Well, time went on and the symptoms changed—as you well know—different things started developing with the dystonia. And I kept saying, she's not doing it any more, she's doing this—such and such—whatever it was. And he said, "That should show you even more precisely that you don't give this type of behavior attention, so she's going on to do something else to get your attention." Okay? Well, Susan was getting progressively worse. In the interim, I was seeing a psychologist every week, Susan was seeing him every week, Marty was seeing . . .

SUSAN'S FATHER: You were seeing him three times a week —we were both seeing him three times a week. Susan was enrolled in a psychodrama class for a year. We were enrolled in a psychodrama . . .

SURGEON: When you say you were enrolled in this, you did it on the advice of . . .

SUSAN'S MOTHER: Positively.

SURGEON: . . . of the psychologist . . .

SUSAN'S MOTHER: Right.

SURGEON: . . . who was trying to help Susan.

SUSAN'S MOTHER: Right. This was the only way—he was treating Susan through us.

SUSAN'S FATHER: He would never discuss Susan. He would only discuss our problems. I'm sure you are aware of what a psychodrama is. We sat with these people who all had marital difficulties.

SURGEON: Had you had any marital difficulties?

SUSAN'S MOTHER: Oh no, but they were coming up.

SUSAN'S FATHER: They began.

SUSAN'S MOTHER: They began—I have to go a little bit further. Then he . . . time went on . . . It's hard to get the right sequence. This was like maybe six, seven, eight months later. Susan was physically absolutely getting worse. She was losing weight. She could hardly move around. You know. One day we got so mad, we took her to an orthopedic doctor. I was the progressive skeptic and mad. Thank God in the end that I was, because I just couldn't accept it . . . I wanted to take her here, take her there, and the psychologist forbade us to take her to any more doctors.

SUSAN'S FATHER: I did. I forbade . . .

SUSAN'S MOTHER: The psychologist did, Fred. You followed through on it. He said if you take her to more doctors, you are just reinforcing her behavior. Well, when we were out with Susan, she could hardly move, she could hardly walk. Fred said, "I'm going to take her to an orthopedic doctor." I mean, her legs were starting to twist, her back arched. And I said, "Thank God. Let's do it." We took her to an orthopedic specialist. He examined her; he X-rayed her from top to toe. He checked the X-rays and he called us and said, "It's very strange. When she is in a prone position, the muscles are all normal and relaxed, and yet when she's in an upright position, all her muscles tense up." And I said, "What is that?" He said, "Well, we don't know, but there's nothing wrong with her. It's probably emotional with her."

SURGEON: That's what makes me so mad. Here's an orthopedist, not a psychiatrist, who sees something wrong. He described what he saw correctly. What he was describing

83

is dystonia. If you put muscles into a gravity position and they antagonistically contract, that's dystonia. That's what he was describing. Furthermore, he said, when asked what was wrong, "I don't know." That's where he should have stopped. He didn't have a clue, so he said it must be emotional! Why? In some cases a psychiatric diagnosis is being made for the benefit of the doctor who can't stand to say, "I don't know."

SUSAN'S MOTHER: This is my point. I don't blame any doctor for not . . . what I think of them professionally for not being able to diagnose it is another story. I don't blame them for not knowing. There are a lot of things that I don't know about housekeeping, and Fred doesn't know about his business. But when they don't know and they won't admit to it and say, "I don't know this. Go to another orthopedic man, go here . . ." They push it off as another emotional thing, because it's just like a wastebasket you throw dirty laundry in.

SUSAN'S FATHER: Let me give you some more. Susan was forced during the first year of her illness . . . We'd planned to send her to summer camp. We asked the pediatrician and we asked the psychologist, and they both said, "Yes, you must send Susan." She was forced to run, to swim, to ride horseback without the use of crutches, of any help whatsoever.

SUSAN'S MOTHER: This was the summer of '69. She wrote the most pathetic letter I've ever read in my life, pleading to come home. She can't stand it. She can't make it to the dining room. She is soaking wet from the strain of getting around. But before she went to camp . . .

SUSAN'S FATHER: The pediatrician, before she went to

camp, the pediatrician signed a normal, healthy, nothing wrong . . .

SUSAN'S MOTHER: And in the note he put, "This child has a very bizarre posture. Disregard. But she's in perfect physical health . . ."

SUSAN'S FATHER: I know Janet. We've heard her mother's story of what they did to Janet. This is the type of thing that someone should be made aware of. We live in an area where some of our neighbors are doctors. And they subscribe to the same books you do. They have a library, but if they would only just read it, or open their eyes for once. These are people who—they know—we're a victim of, how shall I put it?—of suburban medicine. Where referrals stay within the community. When we were finally referred to a neurosurgeon, he was in the community, too, and worked with the neurologist who had said nothing was wrong after he'd examined her neurologically twice.

SUSAN'S MOTHER: Oh, more than twice. More than twice.

SURGEON: When was this?

SUSAN'S FATHER: During her progressive stages.

SUSAN'S MOTHER: In the beginning, and again when she got so bad—we took her back again—we kept running back . . .

SURGEON: We're well into '69 now . . .

SUSAN'S MOTHER: Right. She's losing weight. She's getting worse. Finally the psychologist said, "It's emotional. I can prove it to you"—you see, I was very upset, and I didn't know what to believe—and he said, "I can give this child sodium pentothal and you will see as witnesses that under the influence of sodium pentothal, she will perform perfectly, and that will prove to you that it is an emotional, psychological problem." Now, of course, we know it wouldn't have proven anything because dystonia doesn't act that way—in sleep she was normal.

SURGEON: Did you tell him that?

SUSAN'S MOTHER: No, I didn't know it at the time.

SURGEON: Hold it for one moment. You had a second cousin . . .

SUSAN'S MOTHER: Yes, I will tell you about it.

SURGEON: When did you become aware . . .

SUSAN'S MOTHER: No one took our family histories in that way. But I'll come back to that—I told him okay with the sodium pentothal—"Do it right now and prove it. Then I'll be satisfied. If I know what it is, then I'll be satisfied." He said, "No, since you're so negative . . ." and refused to do it. We went back to the neurologist who had sent us there, and he said, "Since the child's under psychologic treatment, there's nothing I can do."

SUSAN'S FATHER: Then I started to get mad at her for not going along with the psychologist.

SUSAN'S MOTHER: It came to quite a head.

SUSAN'S FATHER: Susan never had emotional problems . . . but we really developed some. Oh boy! Did we!

SUSAN'S MOTHER: This is what happened. We had gone on for about a year, and then the psychologist changed his story. I mean, it was already quite an extreme situation to get attention, and it was getting pretty bad. Then he said . . . he gave me all these books to read on how to raise your child and child management, and all this garbage . . . and he said, then he changed his story. . . . He talked to my husband and said, "You're all right. As far as your part in the family . . ." I had always thought that he was the culprit because he was very strict, with his European background and all—our kids are very well behaved—we were considered oddballs. But that's incidental. Then he said that I was the one—"You're the one, you're doing this to her, because you are so worried about what people are saying, and you demand perfection, and this child is cracking under your pressure." It's true, though, I was worried about what people thought—we were getting quite a reputation in the community. Children were not allowed to play with Susan—there was not a child in our house for almost two years because their parents thought she was a "nut." I mean, this kid was pretty odd, pretty badly shaped, tremors with the head shaking, the whole bit, seeing a psychologist constantly—so they didn't want their kids around her. Up to that point, she'd been president of her class . . . she'd been everything.

SUSAN'S FATHER: You've seen Susan. I'm a proud parent, but I think Susan is a pretty levelheaded kid.

SUSAN'S MOTHER: I kept saying, "It doesn't make sense to me. If she was breaking down this much, how come I haven't heard a word from the school? Her work was beautiful—all A's and B's—teachers were crazy about her." Well, the psychologist resumed, "That just shows that it's you—you're not with her in school. She only does it at home . . ." Which wasn't true—she was just as twisted at school.

You see, this was the start of our problem, because I was very depressed, very down, I had a bad situation going. The doctor kept saying that I was the one who was doing this. Therefore my husband started to get down on me.

Well, one day—I'll give you an example—Susan wears bangs, and I had tried to trim them one day. In order to cut them straight, she had to sit very still. Obviously, at this time that was an impossibility for this child, and she was straining so hard to try and sit still, you know, she knew she upset me with all these things going on. Well, she couldn't stop. She just collapsed on me on the bathroom floor. I thought she had dropped dead or something —she was out cold.

Because her condition was so grave, I was able to get a doctor to come to the house. Before he came, I dragged Susan to the sofa in the living room. He was there in about ten minutes, and her leg was just shaking—it was really going. And he checked Susan and said, "I don't know what happened, but she's all right now. I don't see anything." I said, "Look at her leg—look what she's doing." He said, "Well, she's a pretty nervous child. Bring her into the office. We'll take some blood tests and run a few more tests that I can't do here."

So I called my sister to watch the other children. Fred wasn't home, so I called his brother to help me—I couldn't lift her. So I took her in there, and they checked her and couldn't find anything. Then he came to the conclusion that she had fainted, that that's what happened. I heard one doctor, who was his partner, say to the nurse, "Boy, that's an odd one. Did you ever see anything like that?" She was so twisted up and everything.

Anyway, to make a long story short, I came home—she was exhausted, as pale as can be—and I laid her down on the sofa in our family room, and I closed the shades so she could rest. So he comes home, Fred comes home, and the shades are drawn and she's lying down. Immediately he asks, "What's going on?" It's Saturday afternoon around one-thirty, and I told him, "Be quiet, don't wake her up, she's fallen asleep." "What happened?" he yelled, really getting worked up. I told him what happened. Well, my husband beat me up. I do not blame him in any way whatsoever. He said, "My God, that man is so right. Look what she pulled on you to get attention. She had two doctors checking her. She had your sister run over to take care of the other kids. She had my brother carry her to the doctor's. Look at what she pulled on you today. Look at all the attention she got."

SUSAN'S FATHER: I opened the shades. I roused Susan up. I chased Susan outside to mow the lawn and then proceeded to . . .

SUSAN'S MOTHER: He called the psychologist and told him what I did, and he obviously told Fred how terrible I was.

SUSAN'S FATHER: You see, I'm a very good instruction-follower. In my business I like to go to those who are qualified in their profession, whether it be legal—attorneys —whatever it may be—the best. Unfortunately, there's not a barometer around to find out who's best. And I sincerely believed that the psychologist had just hit everything right on the button—that Susan was like this because . . . people do irrational things under stress.

SURGEON: Had you ever hit your wife before?

SUSAN'S FATHER: No.

SUSAN'S MOTHER: I sincerely believed that the psychologist was doing all this in good faith. No, he had never hit me before—we'd never had an argument in our lives. We'd been going together since we were fifteen . . .

SUSAN'S FATHER: We are going on our sixteenth anniversary this year.

SUSAN'S MOTHER: This was so different . . . This was not our life pattern. When he did it, he was more upset than I was, because I could understand why he was doing it. Then he would come home and I was depressed, and I had quite good reasons to be depressed. He would be angry because I was depressed—it wasn't fair to the other kids. The vicious circle began.

SUSAN'S FATHER: Anyway, what happened—let me make the story shorter—because these are repetitive things, I'm sure . . .

SUSAN'S MOTHER: I could give you a hundred instances . . .

SUSAN'S FATHER: We quit voluntarily ourselves. My wife and I came to the decision that we were not going to go seek any more psychological help.

SURGEON: When did you come to that decision?

SUSAN'S MOTHER: January of 1970.

SUSAN'S FATHER: We decided the hell with it.

SURGEON: When was the episode when you slugged her?

SUSAN'S FATHER: In October of '69.

SURGEON: And what happened to your marriage during that period?

SUSAN'S FATHER: Well, there wasn't any. I was looking for other girls—I never found any . . .

SUSAN'S MOTHER: You weren't really looking for any,

90

Fred. He'd just walk out of the house. Which was more than understandable. He just couldn't take it. I mean, the man worked all day, he came home to a child who was —God knows what. I was in a terrible state.

SUSAN'S FATHER: I was mean to Susan. They kept telling me she could walk, and she pleaded with me for help and I never gave it to her.

SUSAN'S MOTHER: I had known my husband for twenty years. We've been through many, many difficult situations, many trying times. I've never witnessed him break down except for the time they told him that Susan had dystonia —not because it was dystonia—that we could have faced, but he broke down because of how she had been treated, how we had treated her, what had happened to our family because of these mistakes. This is why he broke down.

SUSAN'S FATHER: They tried to make me relive . . . I was six when I came here from Germany, from the concentration camp, my mother was in another one . . . our family was split up all over Germany.

SURGEON: But you all survived?

SUSAN'S FATHER: My brother survived, my mother and father—the rest of them died in there. They tried to make me relive that—in these psychoiogical sessions. That this was where all the antagonism stems from. They tried to get me back there. They tried to make me relive things that really . . . that part of my life was mean and bitter, but it was over with. I didn't carry it with me. I never have. But they tried . . . Susan fell down once in the middle of a crowded street—we were going to a restaurant. The psychologist had said, "Don't touch her if she falls." So I

91

left her lying there and she was almost run over by a bus.

SUSAN'S MOTHER: Well, there are many stories. I nearly killed myself. I came close . . .

SUSAN'S FATHER: I can tell you one fact of life that was true. During this time my wife conceived. Even though we were mad at each other, we weren't *that* mad. She conceived. And she had an illegal abortion—at that time there was nothing legal about an abortion. I had to find an illegal abortionist because she would not have a child knowing that she was an unfit mother. Not to prevent any more mistakes. At the same time I had a vasectomy—also illegal. It was the right thing to do, but we did it for the wrong reason.

SURGEON: How many children do you have?

SUSAN'S MOTHER: We have two others—one's twelve and one's six—and so far they're fine. But let me tell you, an illegal abortion is a rough one. You know Dallas. My husband dropped me off, with the money. . . . When I think about it now, I get the shakes. At that time I was so desperate . . . I even started to think about killing myself. It must have been during the winter, like around December of '69. Susan had to catch a school bus. It was like the equivalent of a half a block, which would take a child maybe two minutes to get to the corner. Well, it took Susan a half an hour because she was crawling at this time. We had to send her to school, and I was the one who had to send her. I had to watch this child crawl down the street, and it was very icy and snowy one morning and bitter cold out, and she left at seven-thirty—the other kids left at eight. And when they all left, I thought, "God, if this is what I can do to another human being, I just don't want to live any longer. Maybe I'll do it to the other kids. And Fred had some sleeping pills, and I took them out and I sat down, and I thought I couldn't take this any more. And I went into the bathroom and I just sat there with them for a while, and that was really close. I don't know what changed . . . I think I thought, "Who will take care of Susan?" I don't know what I thought . . .

SURGEON: What did Susan say all this time? Did she accept the thought that it was . . .

SUSAN'S FATHER: She never thought she was crazy.

SURGEON: They didn't actually say to you that she was crazy?

SUSAN'S FATHER: No, that's a crude way of putting it. But they kept telling her that if she wanted to, there was nothing wrong with her physically—"If you want to sit straight, you can; if you want to walk . . ."

SURGEON: What did she say?

SUSAN'S MOTHER: I think she just kind of held it in. She felt very bad because she knew she was upsetting me, which upset her. She knew that she was the cause of all these things in the family and there was nothing she could do.

SUSAN'S FATHER: The worst thing to her, for instance, about the trip to New York to see you—it wasn't the operation itself—it was seeing the psychologist in your group, because she associates all . . . I mean, she's afraid something's going to change your mind about operating. That you're going to say, "No, Susan, we're wrong. It isn't physical . . ."

SURGEON: The only reason he's examining her is because it's important to have an objective assessment of each patient's intellectual and emotional status before he or she undergoes brain surgery. This helps us in many ways. First of all, it helps us to understand the patient better, and also to appraise the function of the brain from all points of view. Secondly, when we perform the same tests after the operation they are important in assessing the effect of the operation itself.

SUSAN'S FATHER: Right, right. She really understands. She is just frightened.

SURGEON: We got to a point that I want to get back to. In January of 1970, by which time, presumably, you both decided not to have any more psychiatric therapy, at least for yourselves. How did you come to that decision?

SUSAN'S MOTHER: I couldn't stand to go there any more. Fred was released because he wasn't causing the trouble. I was the troublemaker. I would sit there and I would say, "I've got to have some kind of help. I can't stand it any more." He'd say something like, "When you're ready for help, you'll get it." I'd say, "Well, what do you want to talk about?" We even had a case worker come to our house and watch us . . .

SUSAN'S FATHER: And live with us . . .

SUSAN'S MOTHER: . . . to see what was going on. Anyway, I couldn't stand it. I would sit there and he would not allow me to talk about Susan—no, me, when I was a child, my relationship with my mother, when I was in school— all that stuff. I couldn't just talk—we used to sit there in silence. I'd say, "What do you want to know? Ask me a question and I'll answer you." "When you're ready, you'll talk." Well, I didn't know what I was being ready for. I mean, this was what was frustrating. I would sit there for forty-five minutes, not saying anything, and I thought, "My God, my husband is paying forty-five dollars for this. I'm sitting across from the man and I'm not saying anything."

Then this thing happened that triggered me off: I noticed that when I picked Susan up from her weekly psychodrama sessions, she was much worse physically than when I took her. They evidently upset her, or the fact that she anticipated, "Gee, Mom expects me to be better after these when she picks me up." I don't know what it was, but I saw the strain in her every time. And we were sitting at dinner one night, and I said, "Fred, I'm not going. You can beat me up, you can do whatever you want, but I'm not going." We must have all been on the same wavelength, because he agreed.

SUSAN'S FATHER: This is the real kicker—we decided not to go any more. My wife had an appointment the next day to see the doctor. I came home early because I wanted to be there when she told him that we were pulling out. We went there. We waited for him. We walked in. I said, "Doctor, that's it. We need a break. We need rest. I'm not pleading poverty, but we see no help for us or for Susan. We're stopping all treatment as of now."

SURGEON: How long had you all been in treatment?

SUSAN'S MOTHER: About a year and a half.

SUSAN'S FATHER: Up to then, when that man told us to be there, we were there. If it were Sunday or Saturday—it didn't make any difference, we were there. Everything was secondary to Susan's or to our family problem. He said, "You're making the biggest mistake. I want you to leave the office and never come back." He took our deci-

95

sion so personally—like it was a personal failure rather than a family decision that we had made.

SUSAN'S MOTHER: He said if she ever needed psychiatric help, not to bring her back to his office. That if we thought she was bad now, we didn't know what's in store for us.

SUSAN'S FATHER: So we left. He billed me for the session, which I paid for because I didn't want any animosity on our part or his part to us. Susan continued to get worse and worse. The pediatrician saw Susan again . . .

SUSAN'S MOTHER: One day Susan was lying on the floor, so bad—I mean she was having spasms, twisting—she just couldn't sit still. This was going back a few months, and I didn't know what to do for her. She said, "Help me, please help me." I called the pediatrician. I got him on the phone and told him what was happening, and he said to me, "I'll send you out a prescription, but this is not going to cure anything. It will take care of it for the moment, but you people better solve your problems in that household," and he sent me some Miltown.

SUSAN'S FATHER: Our pediatrician is in group practice. That's special, right? So we paid attention when they said something. And they kept referring to Susan as not being physically ill. Anyway, she began to get worse and worse and worse. The more the pediatricians saw her, the more they got fed up with us and Susan. Finally, they said they wanted Susan to be admitted as a psychiatric patient to a children's hospital, affiliated with a medical school.

SUSAN'S MOTHER: They finally came to the conclusion that we weren't making any progress. She had lost about thirty-five pounds.

SUSAN'S FATHER: She was bad. She was on the verge of everything. She was just tragic.

SUSAN'S MOTHER: I knew if this child got one more bad cold, it was doubtful that she would survive.

SUSAN'S FATHER: We took her to this children's hospital, and we saw . . . at the psychiatric clinic there, you see, it's a nonpaying clinic . . . you have to go through the clinic, you can't just walk in as a patient service. It's a state service, I think. The case worker saw her and she almost flipped. She was a young girl, she called in . . .

SURGEON: Was she a psychiatrist?

SUSAN'S FATHER: No, she was a case worker.

SUSAN'S MOTHER: You know, they have to get certain background.

SUSAN'S FATHER: She went out and was back in two minutes with the psychiatrist . . .

SUSAN'S MOTHER: You see, we wanted her admitted, and she said, "I must have a doctor to admit her—as a case worker I can't admit her to the hospital." So she got the psychiatrist who was on duty who could have admitted her. The psychiatrist came in—this man, I'll never forget him—and he looked at Susan, and he read over what we'd told the girl. He took Susan aside—he must have been gone for about five minutes. He came back and said, "There's nothing emotionally wrong with this child. She's the most stable kid I've ever met." He wasn't the one we were originally sent there to see, but he said, "I want this child admitted as soon as possible to the medical division of this hospital, not the psychiatric." The next morning we brought her in . . .

SURGEON: But meanwhile, when he said that there was nothing wrong psychiatrically with this child, how did you react to that?

SUSAN'S MOTHER: I was just dumbfounded.

SUSAN'S FATHER: We were actually pleased because at least it would mean getting her into the hospital. Up until then, we really didn't know if they would admit her at all.

SUSAN'S MOTHER: We were so desperate to get her into some hospital—I think if anybody in the street had offered to take her off our hands, I would have been relieved!

SURGEON: You mean, at that point you just wanted to get rid of her?

SUSAN'S MOTHER: I just wanted to know what I could do with her at that minute. We brought her in the next morning. Then they started taking a case history. The first time in this whole thing.

SUSAN'S FATHER: Actually, later on we found out that there was one doctor who knew what Susan had the whole time. Our family is plagued by hay fever and allergies. This happened to be the allergist. He was a pediatric allergist. He had seen Susan. He had seen our other children, and they were all in for shots. And one day . . .

SUSAN'S MOTHER: No, no, excuse me, Fred. We were going to an allergist, and then this other doctor whom I had known from another area, moved his office out there, so I wanted to switch back to him. So his procedure when a new patient comes—he takes a brief history. He gives a blood test, routine things like that, and he said to me, "Why does your daughter walk like that?" You see this was very early, going back near the beginning. Well, I got very adamant about it, because I was not supposed to discuss it with anybody. So I said, "Oh, that's all right, we know." . . . these were my very words . . . "Don't bother about that, we know all about it, and she's being treated." Then he saw that I was very upset about this. I did not want to discuss it with him, so he wrote on his little card, you know, on his little notes, and he put them away. Well, Susan's allergy treatment was more or less finished, she didn't need shots any more. Then I was back there about two years later with our other children. He said, "How's Susan?" And I said, "Well, she's not doing too well. We're taking her to New York; we hope for an operation." He asked, "What for?" And I said, "We just found out she has dystonia." He said, "You told me two years ago you knew what was wrong with her and you were treating her. What were you treating her for?" I said, "Well, we were told she had emotional and psychiatric problems." And he said, "Sit down for a minute," and he got out Susan's card in a little folder and said, "Here, I want you to look at this." And there was the date on it, and it said, "Dystonia?" Now if I hadn't reacted the way I did, perhaps I would have found out and have been enlightened then and there—two years before. Now if he saw it—he's an allergist—why didn't a neurologist?

SURGEON: Let's go back now to the hospital. You've had her admitted to the medical service. They started to take a history . . .

SUSAN'S FATHER: They immediately found out what she had—in fact, an intern diagnosed it. He had just been studying it. He caused such a furor at the hospital that they stopped operations for an entire day. Well, I'm dramatizing a little. They were so infuriated that this child had been put through what she had because no one could diagnose it.

SURGEON: Who actually diagnosed it?

SUSAN'S MOTHER: The intern. First he took the history, and the next day he told us what it was.

SURGEON: When did you find out that your cousin also had dystonia? Had you known that before?

SUSAN'S MOTHER: No. This is what happened. You know in case histories how they always ask how many brothers and sisters, who's living—somehow it came out. "Did any of the children in your family have any serious illnesses or die at an early age?" And it dawned on me that I had a first cousin who died when he was ten. I was young then, and you know when a child dies, it's not something you discuss with the other children in the family. And there was a divorce in that family, but before he became critical, so I had no contact . . . Then he asked, "Do you know what this child had?" And I said, "No, I don't."

SURGEON: No one had ever asked you before?

SUSAN'S MOTHER: No one had ever asked us anything. Why we weren't even in the category of physical illness. When I found out what it was, I started digging, and finally I tracked down my ex-aunt-in-law. I called her up—I hadn't talked to her in over twenty-five years. I said, "Our daughter is very ill. Please tell me what Jackie died of." She said, "He had dystonia musculorum deformans." And I said, "That's what my daughter has."

SUSAN'S FATHER: The next day they had a seminar about Susan. They took movies, they called all the staff in, all the interns in—they had a rotating service that day—and

they had a seminar on the complacency of modern medicine.

SUSAN'S MOTHER: Their point was that doctors were
shrugging off physical things because they didn't know
what it was. Because at the same time, they had a girl
from Argentina or somewhere who had been in a mental
institution, and they found out she had like a clot or tumor
or something in her brain.

SUSAN'S FATHER: They assigned a neurologist to Susan,
and then sent her to another hospital where there was a
specialist who was using L-Dopa. Well, it turned out that
the doctor and my wife had gone to high school together
and had known each other very well.

SUSAN'S MOTHER: He was telling us what Susan had,
what could be done. Then he said, "Of course there is
surgery." And I said, "Surgery!" I brightened up. I said,
"Why didn't you say that?" Well, the way his tone was
. . . like "This is the last resort" . . . and I figured . . .
I remember I read a book once about a mental institution
where they gave people lobotomies, and they just sat
around and I thought, you know, this must be what it is.
Truly a last resort. Then he said, "Yes, it's done in New
York . . ."

SUSAN'S FATHER: So we called a neurosurgeon who is a
friend of ours practicing in New York. You see, once we
knew what it was, we knew what to do.

SUSAN'S MOTHER: So we called him and said that we just
had the diagnosis that Susan had dystonia, and I wanted
to know more about it. I didn't understand it and I wanted
to know more about it. He kind of explained it to me and
the type of surgery and everything, and he said to me, "If

101

you decide to do it, call me back, and I can make the arrangements for you." Well, it was just kind of hanging. In the meantime, Susan went to visit her grandmother in Dayton, just as a change for her. She flew down there and flew back with somebody. We hadn't seen Susan for about a week, while she was there, and we picked her up at the airport, and when I saw her after not seeing her for a week, it was an absolute shock to me. Not that she had gotten worse in the week, but I was living with it so much day to day, minute to minute, I didn't realize how very bad she was. And we came home from the airport, and she was unpacking her little suitcase, and Fred was working on the lawn, and I walked out the door. I said, "Fred, you can do whatever you want, but I'm taking her to New York." And he said, "Okay."

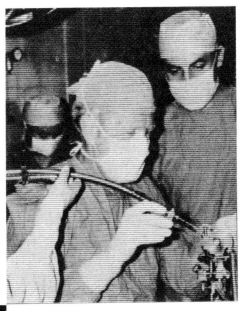

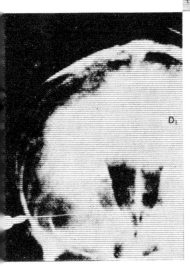

CHAPTER 7

Wednesday 4:00 P.M. The surgeon once again was seated next to Janet's bed. At about two o'clock, Janet's mother had come back to his office and said that Janet had reached a decision and was now anxious to talk to him.

SURGEON: Hi, Janet. Your mother told me you wanted to see me.

JANET: I'm sorry I was such a pest this morning, Doctor —really I am. I hope you're not mad at me.

SURGEON: No, honey, why should I be mad at you—I'm here to help you. I couldn't be mad at you.

JANET: You know, Doctor, that's the first time I've seen you smile.

SURGEON: Well, Janet, I smile often, but I guess most of the time at the hospital, we're preoccupied about something, or thinking about the next thing to do, or worried about someone, and we really don't smile as much as we should. Everyone really should smile in the hospital—of all places. Doctors should smile more, the nurses should smile more, the janitors should smile more—and maybe we should hire people whose only job is to walk around and smile at the patients. It probably would do them a hell of a lot more good than most of the things we do for them.

JANET: I'm really sorry about the way I've been acting.

SURGEON: Well, let's forget about that, Janet, and let's talk about you and why you're here, and let's decide what we'll be able to do about it. Okay?

JANET: I'm here because I have dystonia. And I want to be operated on for it, and I want my arms and legs straight so I can sit up and walk. I want to go back to school.

SURGEON: Well, Janet, before we get to that—which I think is just great and it's just what I want to help you to do—I want you to tell me a little more about yourself. And then I want to explain to you what the operation means, and how you'll have to help me, and what the chances are that the operation will help you. Okay?

JANET: But I've already decided. I want the operation.

SURGEON: Janet, I know a lot about your history, that is, how you were well until you were seven, and then your foot curled up and gradually got worse, but I'd like to know a little bit about you personally. What do you think about?

JANET: I think about getting well. I want to get out of bed.

SURGEON: Okay. Janet, you're crying again. Why are you crying? Are you having pain? Or are you frightened? Why are you crying now?

JANET: I'm scared.

SURGEON: What are you scared about?

JANET: I'm scared about the operation.

SURGEON: Well, honey, that's fair enough. But I'll explain all that to you, and maybe you won't be so scared. It really isn't so bad, and there's a good chance it will help you. Janet, what do you think was the worst part of your illness?

106

JANET: When they locked me in a room. And it was all bare. And just put my food inside the door. And I crawled along and leaned against the wall to get my food. Otherwise I didn't get fed.

SURGEON: Oh, you mean when you were in the psychiatric hospital?

JANET: Yes.

SURGEON: What do you think about the psychiatric treatment that you had, Janet?

JANET: That was murder-hell!

SURGEON: Murder-hell? Why?

JANET: Because I had to crawl on the floor to get my food.

SURGEON: You mean, you literally had to crawl?

JANET: Yes.

SURGEON: How long did that last?

JANET: Until Mom and Dad took me out.

SURGEON: How long were you in the room?

JANET: Almost three months.

SURGEON: Janet, did you think your problem was psychological?

JANET: No.

SURGEON: What did the psychiatrist say to you?

JANET: He said I was wacky.

SURGEON: Well, now, Janet. The psychiatrist didn't just come up to you and say, "Janet, you're wacky." What kind of wackiness did he say you had?

JANET: Up here in my noggin. (Trying to point to her head.)

SURGEON: And what did you say to that?

JANET: I said, *"Phooey!"*

SURGEON: Did you really? Did the psychiatrist ever sit and try to explain to you what your problem was?

JANET: No.

SURGEON: When you were finally sent here, was it because you kept raising hell all the time? You were certainly raising hell when you came here. What have you been thinking about? Did you think you'd ever get better?

JANET: Yes. The doctor in Idaho finally told me about the operation, and I believed him.

SURGEON: But how about before that? When you were in the hospital. Or just lying back at home.

JANET: Then I didn't believe anything. I thought I'd never get better.

SURGEON: What did you think about then?

JANET: I wanted to die.

SURGEON: Did you really, Janet? Being just a little girl, did you understand what that meant? (Janet nods.) And here you are—kind of optimistic.

JANET: Well, I believe it now.

SURGEON: Okay, Janet. Let me tell you a little bit about your disease. As you know, all of this trouble you've been having is a disease called dystonia musculorum deformans. It's not a very common disease, but I've seen almost four hundred other kids that have had it, so it's not exactly that rare, either. You know what it's like, because you've lived with it for four years. Everybody that has been around you knows what it's like, because it's visible and they can see it. They can see your foot twist, or your arm twist, or your head turn, or your back arch, so there's not much I can tell you about that. I can tell you that I'm fairly certain it's not due to any psychological cause. It's not hysterical, and it's not in any way your fault that you have it.

Even though you were born normal, you had some cells in your body that didn't develop normally. They make your brain send messages to your muscles that are not correct, and then the muscles twist and turn and make your arms and legs take on these awkward positions. It's the muscle cramps that give you so much pain sometimes. So the problem is not in your arms and legs, and it's not in your mind psychologically—it's somewhere in the cells of your brain. It's probably due to some error of chemical transmission. Do you know what I mean? In the nerve cells of the brain. So it's into the brain we have to go to try and correct it. Since it's chemical—at least I think it is—I'm sure that someday there'll be medicine that will cure it, or at least the symptoms. We used to have to do the same type of surgery to stop the spasms of Parkinsonism, but there's a drug, L-Dopa, which makes surgery unnecessary most of the time.

The doctors have already tried everything available at the present time which might help you, so the only thing we can do is to operate on your brain to try to balance all of the different parts of it that help to control your movements and the position of your arms and legs.

JANET: Why did the doctor keep telling me I was wacky?

SURGEON: Well, Janet, there are lots of reasons for that, and I'll try to answer you as honestly as I can. One important reason is that illnesses that are caused by some problem in the nervous system—particularly from the brain—are extremely complicated. And since the brain is locked away in a hard skull, we can't get at it or study it easily, and therefore a lot of these illnesses are not well understood. And in addition, many of them get much worse when the patient is upset. For instance, a patient has shaking which is due to an honest disease of his brain, but if he gets emotionally upset—let's say he gets angry with his wife, or his wife gets angry with him, or he's watching an exciting movie, or he gets bad news about the stock market—his shaking will get much, much worse. Therefore, many of the people around him—and sometimes even his own doctor—think that the shaking is due to a psychological condition, but it's not. The shaking is due to some improper function of the brain, and it gets worse when he's upset and his brain is functioning in a more active way and stimulating the part of his brain that is producing the shake. So one of the reasons that the doctor might have thought your problem was psychological was because it was worse when you were upset, and he could see that.

Another reason Janet, is a very human one, I think, and it's a mistake that doctors have been making for centuries. They find it difficult to say to a patient or to a patient's family that they don't really know what the hell is going on. And doctors who go to grammar school and high school and college and medical school, and then take specialty training for five or six years—well, after putting in about twenty-five years getting educated as doctors, many of them can't really believe that there's much they don't know. Of course, there are people who seem to be paralyzed sometime and they're really hysterical—kind of paralyzed with fear—and their problem *is* psychological. And there are some people who twitch all over because they are nervous, and their problem *is* psychological. So therefore, if a doctor has never before seen a patient with dystonia or a kid who twitches all over because something is wrong with his brain, he can't explain it to himself, and he just assumes that the patient is nervous or has some deep, hidden psychological problems.

JANET: I think *that's* wacky!

SURGEON: Well, it may be wacky, but that's how it happens. And in your case, I don't agree that the problem was psychological, although I do think that you may have developed some psychological problems, like pouting too much, or trying to manipulate your mother a little bit too much, or wanting attention every single minute, because of the fact you've been so sick. But that's something to talk about another time.

There's one other thing, Janet, that has to be said about this confusion about organic problems being treated psychologically. That is, that the same mistake is very often made in reverse, even though doctors try to avoid it. Many times operations have been performed upon persons whose real trouble was actually emotional distress, rather than an organic disease which the surgeon suspected. There are lots of patients who go to doctors' offices with pain in their tummies that's really caused by nervousness or worry or even more complex emotional problems. Sometimes, surgeons believe that the problem is actually in the abdomen, and the patient is operated upon. Sometimes we see patients who have been operated on four or five times, and no organic cause is ever found. In some of these cases, the cause probably was up in the patient's noggin, while the surgeon was looking for it inside her abdomen or somewhere else. These are human mistakes, because doctors are

111

human. We all just have to try harder, somehow, not to make them.

JANET: Well, okay, I understand all that. But how about my operation?

SURGEON: Okay, Janet, here's the story about the operation. As I said, we've learned that there are certain areas in the brain which contribute to the neurologic mechanisms that get out of order and that make your arms and legs twist. We don't even know if these are the areas that are diseased, but we've learned that by going in and destroying small parts of them, in some cases, the twisting will stop. And your arms and legs can be useful again.

JANET: Is it dangerous?

SURGEON: Janet, from a statistical standpoint it's not especially dangerous—not as dangerous as letting your disease go on, doing nothing. There is a risk of about two percent that something quite serious can happen to you from this operation.

JANET: At this point, that's nothing!

SURGEON: I've already explained all of the risks in detail to your mother, and we've agreed also that the risk of letting your disease get any worse is probably much greater. I also have to tell you this: that one side of the brain controls the opposite side of the body, and therefore we have to operate on one side of your brain to try and stop the involuntary movements and the torsion and twisting on the opposite side of your body. Then, if that's successful, about three to six months later we do the same thing to try and correct the other side of your body.

JANET: Oh, I know all about that. Susan's told me about

112

it, and she's already been operated on three times and she doesn't mind it.

SURGEON: No, I know she doesn't, but I want you to understand exactly what it is we face, because once we start, then I think we should forge ahead and keep going, even if it takes six operations, unless we get to a place where you're better, or I think we can't do any more. Okay? Now there's one other thing that's necessary, Janet, and that is that the operation has to take place while you're awake.

JANET: I know that, and Susan told me that it hurts. That's why I'm scared.

SURGEON: Well, it certainly isn't the most pleasant thing in the world to go through, and I can see why you'd be scared, because I'm scared every time I have to go to the dentist, but it's the way it has to be. And it really doesn't hurt a lot for several reasons. First of all, the main part of the operation is on your brain, and the brain, even though it's the center of all of a person's feelings, can't feel anything itself. So we can operate on the brain without you knowing it or feeling it, so that won't hurt. And when we make a tiny opening in your head so we can operate on your brain, you can't feel that either. That just makes a little bit of noise when we do it, but it doesn't hurt. So the only thing that does hurt is what we do to your scalp, because the skin is sensitive and that can hurt. Now there are two things we have to do: one, we have to put your head in what we call a "head-holder," so that it will be absolutely still and stay in the same position all through the operation. And we do that by putting four clamps on the side of your head once you're lying on your side on the operating table. So that they won't hurt, we have to inject procaine, or local anesthesia, into your scalp, and you do feel the pinpricks when we put in the local anesthesia, but after that there's no more pain.

What you will feel, and what Susan has probably told you about, is the fact that these clamps are exerting pressure against your skull to hold your head in place, and you'll feel that pressure and it's a little bit uncomfortable, but we've done it hundreds of times to kids and thousands of times to grown-ups, and it really is not that bad. I'm sure you can do it.

JANET: Okay. I told you I'd decided already.

SURGEON: I know that, Janet. The only other thing that can hurt is the tiny incision we have to make in your scalp in order to go ahead with the operation, and there, too, we have to inject some local anesthesia, and what you feel are the pinpricks. So you'll feel about a half a dozen needle sticks when we're injecting local anesthesia, and you'll feel the pressure of the clamps of the headholder, and you'll get a little uncomfortable in one position on the operating table. But aside from that, it won't really be so bad. And I'll be talking to you the whole time, and if you do have some pain or some fear, or if there's something you want to know, all you'll have to do is ask me.

JANET: Doctor, do you have to shave my hair all off?

SURGEON: Yes, Janet, this time I'm afraid we will. Sometimes we can get by with taking just a little bit off, but not with the first operation. But you can get a wig, or else you can start a new style—a new baldy style.

JANET: Okay, Doctor. When do we do it?

SURGEON: Well, Janet, tomorrow's Thursday and I'm going to operate on Susan, so we'll do you on Friday. Is that okay?

JANET: Yes—it's not the thirteenth, is it?

SURGEON: No, honey, it's lucky Friday.

JANET: Okay, Doctor, let's go. And I'm glad you smiled at me today.

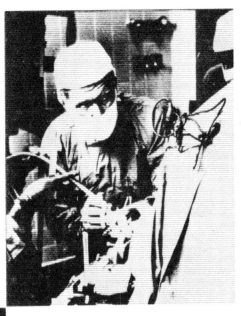

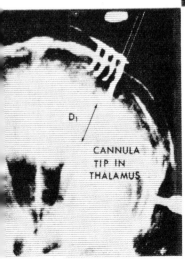

CHAPTER 8

The image that the surgeon would like to have of himself, and that he wishes his patients, residents, and operating-room assistants would have, is one of cool detachment. An operating room cannot ultimately function for the patient's welfare if this role is not established and maintained. But there are times when the burden of responsibility seems overwhelming. The operation has become routine: it is one of thousands just like it, accomplished technically with ease. The patient, however, is unique, and the risks of his life, his functions, his hopes are relived, entered into, each time by the hospital staff and especially by the surgeon.

Sometimes it is impossible to express the crushing, totally exhausting experience that the operating room can be, even though he'd done similar procedures thousands of times before.

He had operated today on a young man who was twenty-six years old and who suffered the spasms of cerebral palsy. He had come from Puerto Rico with his parents. He had violent involuntary movements on both sides, and his speech was barely intelligible. He was intelligent enough to go through college in Puerto Rico, taking a degree in humanities, but now was so totally disabled that he had not been able to work or to care for himself.

Because of the family's financial situation, both the surgeon and the hospital had waived all fees and costs. His parents, distinguished, handsome people, who had spent their lives taking care of him, were laden with anxiety and tension. For twenty of his twenty-six years, they had revolved as satellites about their only son, locked into a filial-centric solar system.

He was examined in detail. There were long discussions outlining the possible risks as well as the possible benefits of the operation. They had been well informed by the referring neurosurgeon and were anxious to go ahead. Please could it be done quickly—could it be done before Friday so they didn't have to live with the anxiety over the long weekend?

He rearranged his schedule, although the week had already been an exhausting one. When he arrived at 7:30 A.M. Thursday, the parents were waiting at the hospital entrance. They told him their son had changed his mind and was so frightened that he couldn't go through with it. So the surgeon went first to the seventh floor and spoke with him gently. Once again he explained that even though there were definite risks to the procedure and he knew how trying it would be, the operation offered the only present hope of alleviating his condition. Since he had come this far, it was worth taking the one or two percent risk of the surgery and trying to face it in order to get some relief from the constant violent involuntary movements. And so the young man agreed. The surgeon came back downstairs and told the parents.

After the patient arrived in the operating room, he started vomiting because of his fear. His head was shaven, he was ready for the operation, but he was throwing up and mumbling in his barely intelligible speech that he didn't think he could go through with it. God, it would have been so much easier on both of them if the patient could have been asleep. But this type of brain surgery requires constant examination of the patient while he is conscious and alert, and unfortunately this young man was not capable of the insight and cooperation of the young dystonics. He was awake and constantly saying that he couldn't go through with it, but then immediately pleading with the surgeon to proceed. The surgeon knew that the young man had come this far and that it was not fair to let him turn back. And so, despite his retching and fear, and while all four extremities and his head and neck were thrashing about, he was placed on the operating table. His head was fixed in the headholder and the operation begun.

By this time he was vomiting violently, which made the operation doubly dangerous, because even in the headholder, the head might move back and forth while the cannula was in the brain. Moreover, an operation that should have taken forty or fifty minutes was prolonged to three hours. All the while, under the drape, the patient kept saying he couldn't stand it, let him up, but then saying, "No—no, continue." By then the surgeon wanted to let him go. On the other hand, once the patient's head was in the holder and the actual operation had been started—the cannula placed—they were both, the young man and the surgeon, committed.

He couldn't let him turn back. But the procedure became one long nightmare. With a sense of constriction in his chest and with a sense of desperation and exhaustion, he again wondered why he didn't stop. Why fight it? Enough, for God's sake, enough. Why didn't he stop? He really didn't know the answer. He did know that he couldn't go upstairs and face it again right at that moment. But an hour from now, there would be Susan. And by that time he'd be ready to start again. He also knew that there were two scheduled for the next day, one of them Janet, and he couldn't bring himself to cancel either of them because they would have to wait over the long weekend, and they couldn't really stand it. Today he felt trapped, tomorrow he might feel exhilarated by it, but today he felt absolutely trapped.

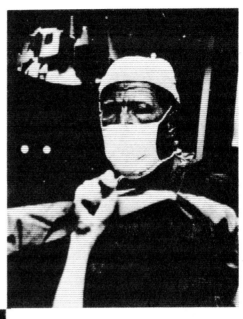

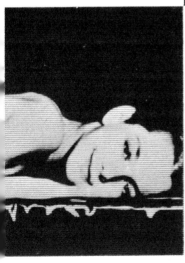

CHAPTER 9

The operating room is large, being about thirty feet square. The table is placed diagonally in the center so that the patient's head is directly under the central X-ray beams, which are twelve feet above and recessed into the ceiling. There is another X-ray beam recessed into the wall, aimed laterally at the side of the patient's head. These will be used during the operation to trace the course of the small, freezing probe that is to be directed into Janet's brain to the thalamus.

Physically Janet and the surgeon are separated from each other by large drapes, from which only the round, shaven top of Janet's head appears, facing the surgeon, who is seated on a high stool opposite it. The scalp has been repeatedly scrubbed with antiseptic soap and gleams under the bright surgical spotlights that are trained on it. The surgeon injects procaine, a local anesthetic, along a line of about two inches of the scalp, where the incision will be made. This is the only anesthesia that will be necessary, since the bone and the brain are insensitive. Janet will feel no pain as the bone is drilled and as the probe enters the soft, gelatinous brain.

On her side of the drape, Janet's head is absolutely rigid, her little face looking up toward the ceiling, as four slender clamps have been placed to maintain her head in an absolutely fixed position. From the shoulders down, however, her body is a writhing, tortured, almost separate entity. Her back is twisted so badly that only her right hip touches the table. The left side of her back is arched and elevated off of the table. Her left leg is so bent that the sole of her foot is pressing flat against her buttock. For more than six months it has been impossible to pull the left leg away from her buttock, and the surgeon has already told the family that he has no idea whether the leg has assumed a permanent, fixed deformity, or whether the leg may relax and be able to be extended if the operation is successful.

Although she is kept awake throughout the procedure, the anesthesiologist is by her side. He is there to comfort her, to ease her anxiety, and to constantly move her legs for her, for they cramp and ache if she tries to lie still more than a moment or two. On his side of the upright green drapery that frames Janet's scalp, the surgeon is flanked, on his left, by his first assistant, a tall, olive-skinned Egyptian who has spent six years training as a neurosurgeon, the last two at St. Barnabas, in order to learn the specialized techniques of brain surgery being employed today for Janet. On his right stands the surgeon's scrub nurse, Peg Ryan. Mrs. Ryan, whose green eyes are constantly filled with concern, appears to take in everything that transpires in the operating room. Throughout the procedure, without a word from the surgeon, she produces whatever instrument is necessary, working with him after all these years like a dancer who knows each step that her partner will make.

Above the operating table, suspended from the ceiling, is a long, narrow mirror, which reflects the tiny twisted figure on the operating table, so that the surgeon can constantly observe not only the patient's head, but also her trunk and limbs which otherwise would be hidden from him because of the drape. Throughout the operation, as the probe enters the brain, and eventually as the target cells are frozen and destroyed, it is necessary for the surgeon to watch the motion of the arms and legs and to speak to the child in order to observe the effects of the operation as it proceeds.

On one of the gleaming tile walls is a large printed sign that says, "Please maintain silence. The patient is awake." The only voices to be heard during the hour-long procedure are those of the surgeon and Janet.

"Okay, Janet, we're all set now, and I'm going to begin. I'll tell you just what we're going to do and when I ask you to do something, or ask you a question, please try to help me and reply."

"All right, Doctor."

First the incision: it is small, about an inch and a half long, on the right side of the scalp, since the operation is aimed at the right thalamus. In general, the right side of the brain controls the left side of the body, and the operation on this day is being carried out to try to disentangle the twisted, cramped extremities on the left side of Janet's body.

Mrs. Ryan hands the surgeon a small, self-retaining retractor, which is placed into the lips of the incision, spreading them about an inch apart and revealing the glistening

127

bone underneath. An electric drill makes it possible to place a dime-size bore hole in the exposed bone in less than thirty seconds.

"You'll hear a whirring noise, Janet, but there won't be any pain, so don't let it bother you, and it will be over in half a minute.

"That wasn't bad, was it, honey?"

"No, Doctor."

"Okay, honey, that's the worst part of it as far as you're concerned and it's over. During the next little while, we'll be doing some things that you won't either hear or feel, and then we'll have to take some X-rays."

A small hook is put into the surgeon's left hand, with which he takes up the dura mater, the fibrous outer covering of the brain, while with his right hand he uses a sharp, tiny scalpel to make an incision in the tented brain covering. About a half an inch of cerebral cortex is now exposed, and with an instrument that looks like electrified tweezers, the tiny vessels on the exposed brain surface are cauterized. This surface is then punctured with the scalpel that was used to open the dura.

"Everything's going along fine, Janet. How are you feeling?"

"My leg hurts, and these clamps are tight on my head."

"I know that, honey, but be patient. We'll go just as quickly as we can."

A slender rubber tube is threaded through the opening in the surface of the brain to a point about two and a half inches below the surface, where it enters a fluid-filled cavity, one of the ventricles of the brain. Ten cubic centimeters of fluid is withdrawn and replaced by equal

128

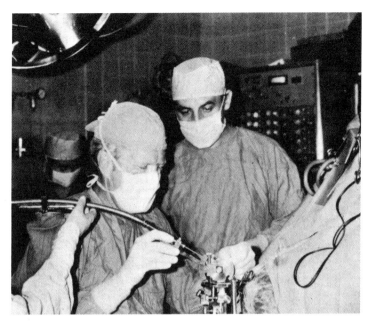

The delicate aiming of the cryocannula toward its target within the brain is begun.

amounts of air, after which the rubber tube is clamped shut. This air will form a shadow on the X-ray plate soon to be taken, and the shadow of the ventricles serves as the landmarks or map by which the surgeon will guide his probe to the thalamus.

Before taking the X-rays, a special instrument, which is called simply "the guide," is attached to the head of the table. This instrument holds the probe as it is being passed into the brain, and helps to direct it in three dimensions, so that its tip can be accurately placed in the surgical target deep within the brain. When the guide has been attached to the table, the probe is placed in it and is aimed toward the thalamus. It cannot enter the patient's brain, however, until X-ray confirmation of its correct aim has been achieved.

"Janet, you'll hear everybody walking around for a few minutes. We're not leaving you, but it's necessary to take some X-rays now, and we all step down to the far end of the room while these are being taken. It then takes about three or four minutes until these first sets of X-rays are developed. After that, it'll only take us ten seconds every time we want to take an X-ray, but this time it takes a couple of minutes longer, so just be patient, and as soon as we have these X-rays we'll be able to move right along."

"How much longer will it take, Doctor?"

"I think it will take about thirty minutes more, Janet."

"I have a bad headache now."

"Well, that's probably due to the air we've just injected, Janet, but it will last only a few minutes and then go away."

Angelo has already placed the X-ray films under and alongside of Janet's head. He moves outside of the room to activate the long X-ray tubes in the ceiling and in the wall, so that within moments two separate views of the air shadows within Janet's brain will be available, and the surgeon can select the target and make certain that his slender probe is accurately aimed at it.

During the few-minute interval while waiting for the X-rays, the surgeon and his assistant and technicians stand by the view box waiting. There is little conversation as the surgeon gazes through the window out over the Bronx. The dust has collected on this window in the scrub room outside of the operating room, and some clever fellow has printed with his finger in the dust, "Wash me!" No one has yet taken this advice seriously, so the surgeon calls it to the attention of the circulating nurse, who runs for a clean sponge to erase the message.

Although the surgeon has stepped to the scrub room a few feet away to view the X-rays, the anesthesiologist sits on a tall stool by the table, holding Janet's hand and speaking softly to her. She repeats that her head hurts, and once again asks how much longer. He moistens her dry lips with a wet sponge, reassures her, and says, "About twenty minutes more, Janet."

Angelo places the X-ray films on the view box, and sterile instruments are handed to the surgeon, including a sterile ruler and a tiny stylet. Quickly the measurements are scratched on the X-ray and the target is marked. The shadow of the probe, still outside of the skull, can be seen on the X-ray film and its direction evaluated. In order to place its tip in the target, within the thalamus, it will be necessary to move the probe three millimeters back and three millimeters to the right. After this, it must be placed 6.5 centimeters (about two and three-quarter inches) below the surface of the brain where it will find its target. The surgeon returns to his stool at the head of the operating room and the corrections are readily made in the guiding instrument.

"Janet, everything looks fine. The X-rays are great. Would you hold your left hand in the air for me? No, hold it a little higher, honey, so I can see it over the drape."

"Can you see it now, Doctor?"

"Yes, Janet, I can see it. Now open your hand wide and

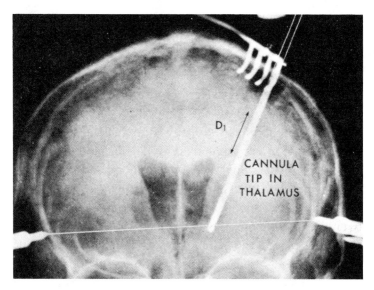

The X-ray confirms the proper localization of the cannula tip within its target on the thalamus, deep within the brain.

try to move your fingers." The arm is raised, but it is twisted, and the fingers are closed in the palm.

"I can't open it, Doctor. It won't open."

"Okay, Janet, just hold it in the air for me, and leave it there for a moment."

The probe is pushed through the tiny opening in the cortex of the brain, and gently advanced centimeter by centimeter, until its tip rests 6.5 centimeters below the surface of the brain.

"Put your arm down now, Janet. That's a girl. Now, Janet, say as loud as you can, 'Around the rugged rock the ragged rascal ran.'" She repeats it in a faint voice, but her pronunciation is good and the quality of her voice is not

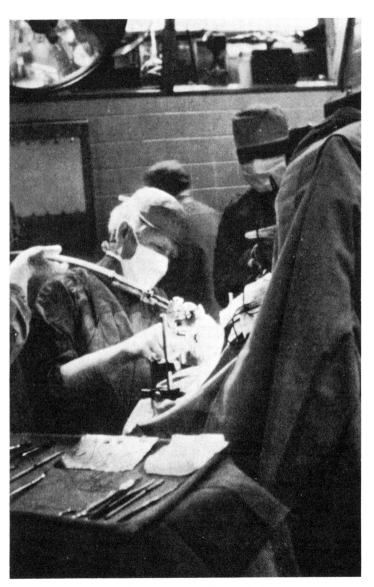

The surgeon advances the cannula slowly into the brain.

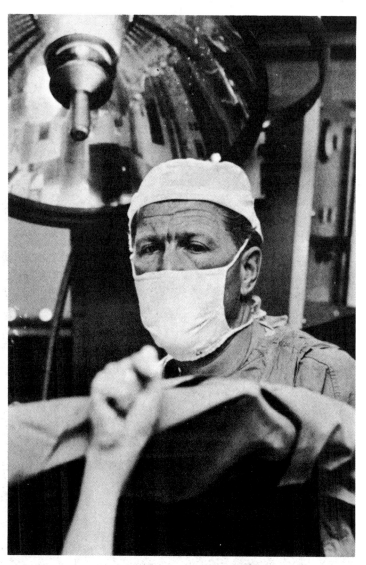

The tiny arm is raised, but the fingers are closed in the palm. "I can't open it, Doctor. It won't open."

changed. Her speech has not been affected by the entry of the probe into her brain, an important sign that has to be followed during this type of surgery.

"Now lift your arm for me again, Janet." The tiny withered arm comes up, still twisted. The thumb and fingers are still involuntarily pushed into the palm. "Can you open your fingers, Janet?"

"No, Doctor, I can't. These clamps are killing me, Doctor. How much longer?"

"About twenty minutes more, Janet. Be patient. It really isn't pain, honey, it's the pressure of the clamps and you're getting a little tired. But the major part of the surgery is over and we just have to get a few more X-rays and then go right ahead."

"X-rays, please." This time the X-rays are taken with Polaroid film and are developed and ready in ten seconds. The stainless-steel, vacuum-insulated, freezing probe is seen within the brain alongside of the air shadows, and the accurate placement of its tip in the ventral lateral portion of the thalamus is confirmed.

The surgeon walks around to the side of the table, allowing his assistant to remain at the head, since he now must personally test the patient as the freezing process deep within the brain takes place.

First he makes an attempt to move the twisted foot away from its superflexed position against the buttock. "Ohhh, stop, Doctor. That kills me when you touch my foot. Please don't touch my foot."

"Okay, Janet, I won't touch it right now, but as you know, the reason we're keeping you awake is to be able to test your leg and your arm during the operation. It's the

135

only way I have of knowing if we're helping you or not, and that's why you've gone to all this trouble of coming to the operating room. If I'm actually hurting you, tell me and I'll stop whatever we're doing, but don't be overly frightened because I won't do anything to continue hurting you. We have to see if we can get your leg down or not."

"I'll try, Doctor."

"Okay, John, minus ten, please." John Orzuchowski, the electronic technician in the operating room, sets the control on the cryogenic surgical system so that liquid nitrogen will begin to enter the freezing probe. Gradually the tip of the probe will assume temperatures far below zero to freeze an area about the size of a large pea. The cessation of function of this small region of the brain, hopefully, will stop the abnormal impulses twisting Janet's arm and leg.

When the temperature has reached minus ten, no change is noted in the arm or leg. "Janet, say 'St. Barnabas Hospital' as loud as you can."

"St. Barnabas Hospital."

"That's good, Janet, your speech sounds clear and maybe even a little bit louder now. Count up to ten for me, dear." She does. "Oh, that's great, Janet. Okay, John, minus thirty, please." When the temperature has reached minus thirty, the fingers and thumb of the left hand have visibly relaxed. "Janet, lift your left arm in the air." This time she does so briskly and the palm is open. "Janet, do you notice any difference when you do that?"

"I think it feels a little looser—and—Doctor, my hand is open! Is it really open?"

136

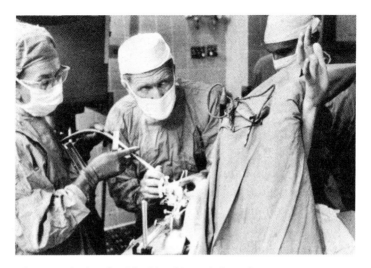

This time the hand is lifted briskly and the palm is open.

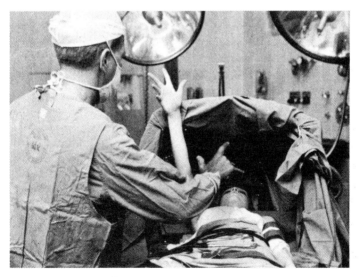

"Try to wiggle your fingers."

"Yes, honey, it's really open. Hold your arm in the air and try to wiggle your fingers, Janet." She does so, and the anesthesiologist and surgeon, the assistant and nurse all look at each other and smile, and some of the awesome tension is relieved. It looks as though things will go along well.

"Okay, John, minus fifty." Then minus seventy. Then minus ninety. By the time the temperature has reached minus ninety, and about two full minutes after the freezing process has begun, the surgeon can hold Janet's left foot without any complaint from her.

"Janet, I'm going to try to extend your left leg a little bit. I've been holding your foot for the last half minute and you haven't said anything, so I assume it doesn't hurt you any more."

"No, Doctor, it doesn't hurt now."

"Okay, I'm going to try to pull it down." The surgeon places his hand on the heel of her left foot, and gently pulls it away from the buttock. The foot comes all the way down so that the leg is now extended ninety degrees from the knee. It had been over a hundred and eighty degrees up against the buttock, with the foot extended almost straight along with the leg. "Janet, can you move your ankle?" The small ankle moves back and forth voluntarily for the first time in more than two years.

"Janet, can you tell that your foot is away from your backside now?" Janet half sobs "Yes"—the tears this time from excitement, not pain.

"We're almost finished, honey, and it looks as though things are going along very well. Minus one twenty, John." The probe is allowed to remain at minus 120° for two min-

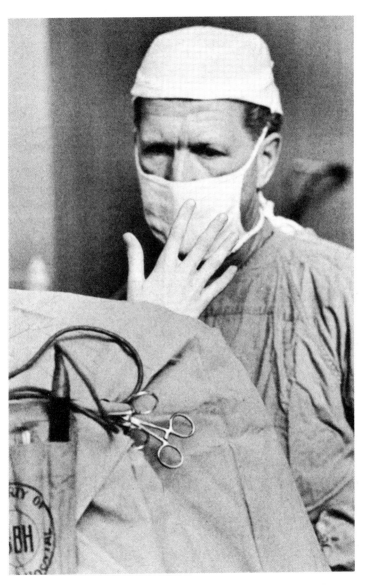

The hand is open. It looks as though things will go along well.

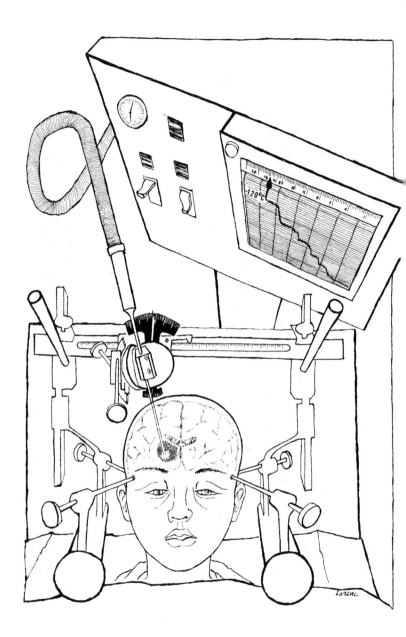

utes. During this time the foot remains away from the buttock and the leg can be almost fully extended by the surgeon.

He turns his attention to the arm now. Placing two of his fingers in the small palm, he says, "Squeeze my fingers, Janet." She does so. "Janet, can you tell that you're now moving your left fingers?"

"Yes."

"Could you do that before?"

"No, Doctor, I haven't moved my hand for a year or more. I—I—I can't believe it!"

The tip of the cannula has thawed and is gently removed. "Janet, the main part of the operation is all over. I'm going to let Dr. Amin put just a few stitches to close up while I run down and tell your mama that everything's okay."

"Okay, Doctor, can I go back to my room now?"

"Just a few minutes, honey, in just about five or ten minutes you can go back to your room. I'm going down and speak to your mother now."

"Okay, Doctor."

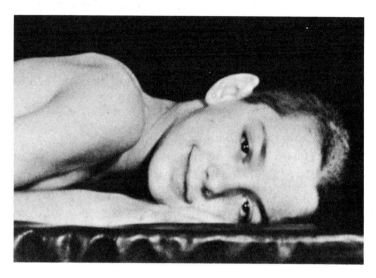

One week after the operation. A smile has returned to a pretty child's face.

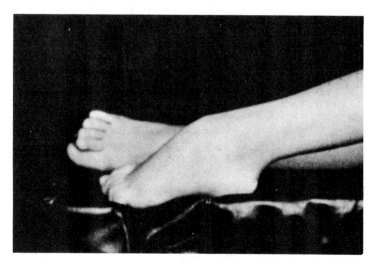

Left foot, right foot. Progress, but still a long way to go.

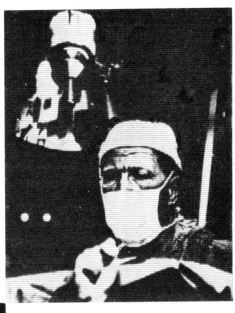

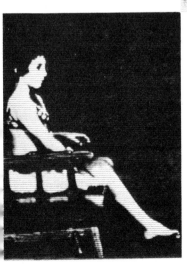

CHAPTER 10

The two operations of the morning, followed by rounds, appointments and consultations were over. Still to come was a talk to be given that evening to a group of divinity students at a nearby seminary. The surgeon sat at his desk and began to look over his speech:

New, seemingly radical surgical procedures, whether they probe sacred recesses of the brain, involve organ transplants from one human to another, or provide artificial means of maintaining the vital functions of life when the patient's own vital functions have ceased, all introduce new moral and ethical dilemmas for both patients and doctors.

Moreover, advances in biologic science that are still at the basic or laboratory stage, such as genetic engineering, computerized tele-transmitted mind control, and drug-induced behavioral manipulation, have raised the possibility of revolutionary changes for good or ill in the human condition. This scientific revolution introduces moral problems as compelling as those produced by the Copernican and Darwinian upheavals. It threatens to remove man as a unique being even further from the center of his own universe. When Gertrude Stein was on her deathbed she imploringly asked those gathered about her, "Tell me, what is the answer?" Since no one could reply, she said, "Well, then, what is the question?" My purpose here is to define the question.

I will not pretend to answer it because it is unanswerable. I shall not be able to provide specific suggestions or any absolute truth that can resolve the question. My hope is that joining the dialogue helps to keep the question open. I am convinced that questions arising from biomedical innovations cannot be addressed without a continuing interdisciplinary exchange that will heighten sensitivity and enlarge the scope of those ultimately charged with the value-judgments that are fundamental to the future of man.

Medical advances often produce new problems that are sociologic and moral as well as medical in nature. The most pressing of these, of course, is the overpopulation of the earth as a result of a lessening of infant mortality and the prolongation of life. This has crystallized the question of abortion as one means of population control and has forced the scientist as well as the theologian to face the question of the right to life.

One paradox resulting from the ability to prolong life is that many have been forced to endure years of helplessness and mental as well as physical suffering as antibiotics, catheters, intravenous feedings, and respirators maintain vital functions that produce only a vegetable existence. This has introduced consideration of a new right—the right to die. Is there ever a time when we should go beyond this and assist the patient to a painless, dignified exit from life?

An area of research that is Orwellian in scope is that of mind control. The search for pharmacologic or neurosurgical or behavioral techniques of relieving mental illness and

146

pain suggest means of pacifying or otherwise controlling the minds of entire populations. Who will ultimately control these techniques?

The most spectacular and revolutionary biologic development is the ability to control human heredity. The ability to change or engineer genes of an unborn fetus holds forth the promise of avoiding many forms of mental retardation and a host of other birth defects. On the other hand, this new exploding science of genetics—which started with discoveries by an Austrian priest, Gregor Mendel, in the nineteenth century, and has evolved into discoveries of the molecular nature of genetic transmitters by James D. Watson and Joshua Lederburg and others in the past two decades—this exploding science carries the ominous possibility of one day cloning, or making exact copies of human beings. Man could create, perhaps, quite a different type of humanity than we now know. Does it violate the meaning of life to technologically change man? The bioethics of the situation are so complex that some scientists have asked their colleagues for a moratorium on this avenue of research until a more systematic means of arriving at value judgments can be developed.

None of these judgments can be attempted unless we are willing to face the fact that each of these questions concerns the very nature of human existence. We must be willing to confront the ultimate question—What is the purpose of life?—if we are to develop ethical guidelines that may determine what we do with it.

Now, it would seem self-evident that no surgical lion in possession of his faculties would presume to leave the domain of his surgical theater and enter the theological arena in order to put his head in the mouth of the Christians by describing the purpose of life. However, this is a problem that has confronted me thousands of times during my career in neurosurgery. Almost daily, in making decisions dealing with human life, the moral judgments are often much more difficult than the scientific or medical questions.

I would like to put these complex philosophical problems in perspective by providing a few illustrations of the ethical dilemmas that arise each time a surgeon makes the awesome decision to allow his patient to assume the risk of any surgical procedure. This dilemma is heightened to some degree in the case of brain surgery since the brain controls not only vital physical functions but also the intellect, the emotions, the personality, and the individuality of the patient. Brain surgery encompasses the possibility of changing the human mind, and thus offers a microcosmic view of the bioethical issues to which I have alluded. Furthermore, brain surgery is a relatively recent art, and as it has assumed an increasingly scientific aspect, many of the operations in this field are new and investigative in nature. Consequently, the question of research on human beings is intricately involved with many neurosurgical procedures being done today.

I should like to cite my own experiences with investigative neurosurgery in dystonia musculorum deformans. Since there is not as yet any drug that can reverse the symptoms of this disease, neurosurgeons became interested in the possibility of lessening the pain and muscle spasms by operating on delicate mechanisms within the brain.

The symptoms of this disease, which are passed along

genetically from generation to generation, have not yet been reproduced in animals. Therefore, new surgical approaches, even though based on experience in the laboratory to some extent, ultimately have to be tried for the first time on a human being.

This brings me, then, to a basic ethical question: how does one decide to operate on the brain of a child, who has a disabling disease, for which there is as yet no cure, for the first time? I was faced with this situation more than fifteen years ago when my neurosurgical experience with other diseases led me to believe that a new surgical approach could relieve some of the symptoms of this disease in children. Naturally, since we had not done this operation before, I could not define the risks clearly. I was not sure what chance this new procedure had for success. It was, therefore, to be an experiment on the brain of a human being. On this occasion the decision was made in concert with the patient and her parents, because of their desperation and willingness to assume any risk since they were overwhelmed by the constant suffering the child had undergone. I, too, was moved to try this procedure for the first time in that child because of the nature of her symptoms.

However, even though in that instance the procedure was remarkably effective, I am not certain that the criterion for making the decision was the correct one. Suppose that first operation had not been successful—or had made the patient worse? I have seen many desperate patients since, willing to undergo any risk for a chance of relief of their symptoms. That single criterion, however, is not enough. Is the possibly erroneous theoretical idea of the neurosurgeon enough? If that first operation had been unsuccessful or had proved harmful to the child, would I have been ethically wrong for trying it? One runs the risk of being very wrong in taking such a step the first time, and the concomitant risk of a burden of great guilt accompanies every decision. Would declining to try be as potentially wrong from an ethical viewpoint?

Once the operation proved successful, since few other surgeons in the world were yet performing it, there was an overwhelming number of patients who sought help in our institution. Physically and economically the institution in which I performed this surgery could not admit everyone who sought help. Therefore, we were often faced with the decision as to who to choose first. What criteria should be employed for deciding that one patient deserved priority in hospital admission for this new procedure rather than another? What could conceivably make one human life any more important than that of another?

One of the many letters we received at that time was from a young man in Hungary, who, despite his progressive dystonic symptoms, had earned a Ph.D. degree in biochemistry. However, by the time he received his degree he had become totally incapacitated by the disease. His letter was moving, intelligent, desperate. The hospital agreed to provide a bed for him, absorbing all costs from their endowment fund, if he could provide his own transportation to this country. He did so, was successfully operated on, and subsequently immigrated to this country. He is now a research professor at a western university and is engaged in cancer research.

It would seem that his possible benefit to society if the operation were successful was a reasonable criterion for choosing this individual. However, one cannot say that his inherent dignity, person, or conscience were more meaningful than that of another who was less educated or less expressive in his application for help. It is impossible to confront this dilemma without actually entering into the suffering inherent in the situation. Paradoxically, in many ways, this makes an ultimate decision even more difficult.

As experience was gained with this procedure, many of my colleagues and I developed new and more ingenious instrumentation for this type of brain surgery. Various types of stereotactic devices—instruments that assist the three-dimensional localization of a probe or electrode or cannula deep into the brain—had already become employed throughout the world. This followed early research by the first brain surgeon of functional diseases, Sir Victor Horsley, in England at the turn of the century, and advances in human stereotaxis by Ernest Spiegel and Henry Wycis and others in this country during the last three decades. Furthermore, new technological methods of destruction of brain tissue, such as the cryosurgical instrumentation that we developed, were invented. Naturally, each of us was anxious to find new horizons for the particular tool he had invented or pioneered.

A great ethical dilemma arises, however, from the urge to use one of these techniques simply because it is there. This sometimes leads to a triumph of technique over reason. Some have expressed just such doubts about cardiac transplantation—that is, using the technique before the central problem of rejection of the organ by the recipient has been solved—simply because the technical maneuver has been mastered.

My own awareness of this ethical problem in human research was heightened a few years ago when I reread the proceedings of an international meeting of neurologists and neurosurgeons of which I was chairman. During the meeting, an eminent professor, one of the most brilliant innovators in modern neurosurgery, and one whose work in this field preceded my own, described a brain operation he had developed. The procedure was long, arduous, and carried considerable risk for any patient subjected to it. In the course of his scientific discourse he said, "We do not advocate nor are we embarking on any therapeutic regime. It is an experiment."

He then outlined the technical difficulties and dangers inherent in the procedure and concluded, "All of this cannot be thought of in any way as a therapeutic procedure." No one at that time, including myself, rose to argue that this type of procedure, performed on a human being by a surgeon who states that it is not a therapeutic procedure, is out of harmony with reason. It is absurd.

Fortunately, in recent years Professor Henry Knowles Beecher, Rev. John Fletcher, and others have heightened our awareness to the point where no one today would make this kind of statement in a medical congress or, it is hoped, would carry out such experiments. One can no longer carry out investigative procedures in humans without confronting the question of what the procedure is for. If it is to test a technique or to suggest that the research has some ultimate value not related to the individual being investigated, it is a phantasmagoria.

As with many so-called medical advances, the development of a surgical procedure introduced new problems which the dystonic patient and those responsible for his care did not have to face in previous years, because there was no satisfactory treatment.

A few of these new problems can be illustrated by the case of a young girl, Nancy, on whom I operated for the first time in 1957, when she was eleven. By that time we already had enough experience to know that usually the operation worked. We also knew that the risk of surgery was not great, but that success was not inevitable. In some cases it had not relieved the symptoms. Nancy had had the disease for four years by the time she was operated on, and she was completely incapacitated. Following two operations, one on each side of the brain, she appeared to have been completely relieved. However, within six months of the second operation her symptoms recurred, and she was again helpless, disappointed, depressed, and seeking help. At that time I did not know whether her young brain could tolerate a third operation of this type. Having been well for a short period, she was more willing than ever to assume the risk of a third attempt. Having had success with this new procedure I had developed, I was unquestionably highly motivated not to give up. But there is some question in this type of surgery, which carries a risk to the human brain, as well as in other vigorous treatments in chronic disease, as to when is the proper time to quit. When might the risk of operating outweigh the possibility of benefit?

I might add parenthetically that I am still grappling with the same question: when is it time to quit? On a few dystonic children, I have operated as often as six times, each time with increasing trepidation. It is difficult to suppress one's willingness to enter into the suffering and hurt in each child's situation, but I would still not be certain what to do if faced with the question, should I operate a seventh time if the sixth has not been successful.

Nancy's physical recovery introduced many new problems. First of all, having been incapacitated and totally without any social life or friends for more than four years, she was quite suddenly well. That is, well physically. Her parents happily sent her off to school, which was virtually a foreign land she had not entered since her illness. She suffered a generation gap among her own classmates and as a result became totally alienated. As an incapacitated child she had been motivated so strongly during her illness that she stayed abreast of her school work by studying at home, but she dropped out of school at fifteen when her sociologic progress could not keep up with the technologic progress of her recovery from dystonia.

This exemplifies the paradox that is often inherent in medical progress: new problems are produced that also become our responsibility. It became necessary to treat Nancy's alienation and her social problems, which were the result of successfully treating her dystonic symptoms. This is not unlike, qualitatively, the medical need to control life on earth as a result of having successfully prolonged it.

Having subsequently successfully managed her social rehabilitation, when she was twenty Nancy and her fiancé came to visit me to discuss the advisability of marriage. This is a right that would appear to belong to the individuals in question, but Nancy was troubled by many problems. Although she had been well by that time for nine years, she lived with a constant fear that her symptoms might come back. When, she asked, could she be free of this fear? The only true answer to that question is never. Should I have allayed her anxiety by saying, "Well, nine years have gone by and so you must be cured by this time"? Or should I have told her quite frankly that we could never really be certain that one day the disease would not return? I chose the latter course.

Should she marry? Suppose she married and her symptoms returned? Would this be fair to her fiancé? These were questions that had to be faced honestly by the two of them.

They did face these questions and did marry, and then returned with the most difficult question of all: could they have a child?

This is the really loaded question. It deals with all of the dilemmas inherent in the problem of ultimate concern. Actually, as is usually the case, by the time the question is raised, the girl's already pregnant. Whether the stress of pregnancy could possibly induce a recurrence of her own symptoms, I did not know. I did know, however, there was a distinct possibility that Nancy's child would carry the gene that had produced those symptoms in herself. Could Nancy bear to wait until the child reached fifteen, and had, more or less, passed the danger point? Could she endure the same nightmare twice in one lifetime? What right did Nancy have to bring into the world a child who would have to live, either knowingly or unknowingly, under the possible threat of one day seeing his or her own limbs contort because of an inheritance that could have been predicted in advance?

What was the right of the fetus, already conceived, to be born? Conversely, did the fetus have any right not to be born, since we knew that there was one chance in four that the child would carry a polluted gene? Would this child someday berate his or her mother for allowing such a birth to happen?

On a broader scale, in an overpopulated world in which one in ten already carries the stigmata of some type of inherited disease, what right have we to further pollute the genetic pool of humanity? It has been postulated that continued production of genetic diseases combined with the population explosion will result in a world which is one gigantic hospital filled with the physically and mentally defective. What role should I play, after relieving these dystonic symptoms in a child, in preventing the passage of this genetic defect to a new generation? Helmut Thielicke in his great work, *Theologic Ethic*, says that an imposed solution to such a problem is anti-ethical and makes of man a mere object. The child itself, he says, once grown, who harbors genetic defects must be brought to understand the need to avoid reproduction probably through sterilization. Do you agree?

I do not know the answers to these questions. I do know that as doctors, we must continue to examine with the humanists, theologians, and with our fellow-men, these questions: What is man? What is the purpose of life? What in the hell are people for?

There are many possible answers; an awareness of the various possibilities will help us to deal with these practical problems more concretely and satisfactorily.

Recently I wrote to a cross section of persons, including former patients, college students, aged pensioners, and long-term chronically ill patients, asking them what they believed to be the purpose of life. Each answer was meaningful. But I have chosen one, from the Hungarian biochemist I mentioned earlier, to exemplify this awareness:

Dear Doctor:

I have received the questionnaire which you sent to me, asking about the purpose of life. I know that you have sent this to many of the patients that you have operated upon, and I would be interested to know what some of the other answers are. It's certainly a difficult question, and my experience of being seriously ill has had a great effect on my answer.

Before you performed the two operations on me, I think my opinion about the purpose of life was completely different. I think at that time I was more selfish and the purpose of life I thought to be more materialistic. I think not only myself, but everybody is trying to find his happiness. This happiness means different things to different people: a new car, a home, money, etc. After my operations, at first, I had to learn to find my place in society because I was separated from others. They looked at me and felt sorry for me. I hated this type of attitude, so I turned back to my work in the laboratory where I tried to find all the things I couldn't find outside. But everything changed, a new world opened up for me after you performed the two very successful operations. After that time, contact with people showed me that the selfish attitude about finding one's so-called happiness does not always lead to the true satisfied meaning of happiness. During this time, and because of you, I think instead of trying to find happiness in individual things, trying to help others find a satisfied life meant a self-satisfaction and happiness for myself. But it doesn't necessarily mean that I am not trying to find my own happiness in my work and in my private life.

Looking back on what I have written, I think the purpose of life means happiness, but this happiness covers a large area. Also I think everybody's opinion about the purpose of life is the same but the approach is different. However, I believe that circumstances can influence different people to find happiness in different things.

Sincerely,

Andros

With Camus, I suggest that the best hope we can offer for the future of man is a permanent dialogue to keep the question open. I suggest that young philosophers, humanists, and priests, should join their contemporaries in the medical sciences—infiltrate the medical schools and hospitals if necessary—to evolve a biomedical ethic that will insure human values within the already vigorous biologic revolution.

Centuries ago, when the purpose of life seemed more apparent, body and soul were consummately cared for by a single person, the witch doctor. The dichotomy of this calling into medical and spiritual specialties has left a void as yet unbridged.

By the time of the Renaissance, Pope Alexander VI was already stating that those least concerned with religion were those most concerned with being at the center of the church. More recently, Rev. Joseph Fletcher wrote, "Moralists who spend little or no time on the terminal wards of a modern city hospital cannot contribute much in the way of realistic opinion or relevance on the subject of euthanasia."

A decade ago, the Surgeon General of the United States Public Health Service, and many other concerned doctors, questioned the judgment of many of their colleagues who were conducting medical research, using ill human beings as their subjects. Rev. Fletcher was correct in urging his students of theology and the humanities to become more knowledgeable about scientific, biologic, and medical problems in order to contribute to the humanization of medical care in the midst of an increasingly technologic society. Conversely, Professor Henry Knowles Beecher, himself an eminent medical investigator, has urged his scientific colleagues to train their students adequately in the sociologic and humanistic aspects of their calling, so that they may be continually aware and conscious of the grave responsibility which they have accepted when they decided upon a medical career.

It is apparent that the future generations of intelligent, informed, conscientious, compassionate, responsible doctors called for by Professor Beecher, who can undertake medical judgments that may possibly violate as well as defend life, must face the question of the nature of existence and its purpose.

Moreover, it is the purpose of each unique man or patient that must be considered. No one considers his own purpose, whether it be to achieve the beatific vision, to support pleasure as the highest good, to fulfill duty, to serve oneself, or to simply exist, as less deserving than any other. An ongoing dialogue of humanists with their medical and scientific colleagues will serve, as Dr. John Knowles has pointed out, each discipline in heightening awareness, enlivening imagination, increasing responsiveness, broadening interest, and clarifying purpose.* In the end it will result in a quickened ethical sense.

Even if this goal so consummately to be desired is achieved, it is justifiable to ask: When will our anxieties about these enormous problems be relieved? When will concrete, absolute solutions be reached? When will the dialogue be over?

If we are really lucky—and work at it hard—never.

---

* *Views of Medical Education and Medical Care,* ed. John H. Knowles, M.D. (Cambridge, Mass.: Harvard University Press, 1968).

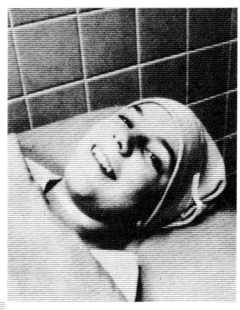

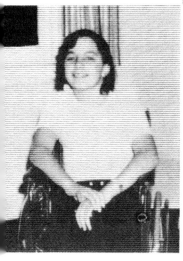

The Months

That Followed

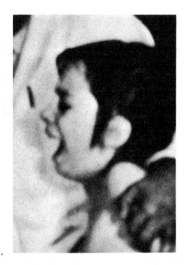

A few months before . . .

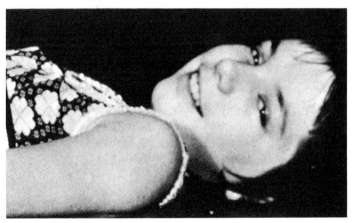

A few months later, thirty pounds heavier, and a broader smile. "I'm better, but I'm still not walking, Doctor. Let's try the other side."

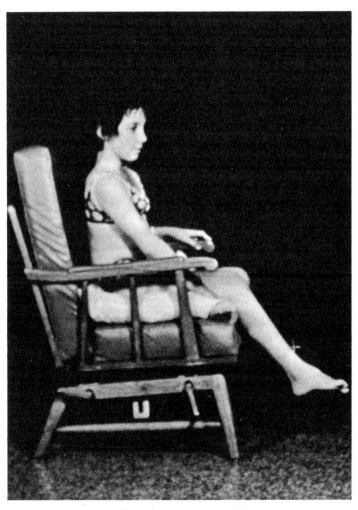

"I can sit. I feel good, but I still want to walk."

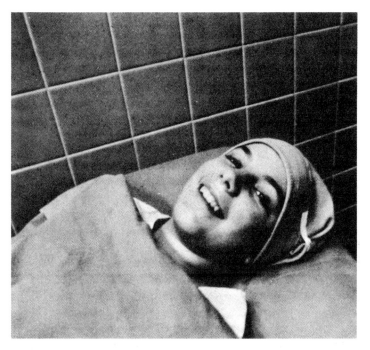

"Well, Doctor, here we go again. Operation number three. I feel like a veteran now. I think I'll catch up with Susan."

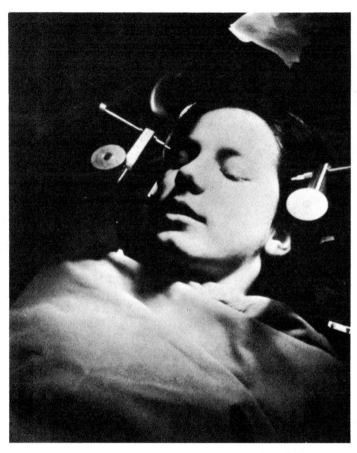

Her head, once again held steady in the viselike grip of the head-holder. Awake, no longer helpless, not quite so lonely, still brave, still hopeful, awaiting preparation for operation number three. Thirteen years old.

Three operations behind her, eight inches taller, forty pounds heavier, arms and right leg normal. Once again an A student, and president of her class. There is still some deformity of her left foot, which prevents her from walking. "Another operation, Doctor. Let's have another operation."

We've come so far, but each new operation carries a risk. Janet's mother and Janet can't wait for the day when she may walk again. The surgeon is cautious, uncertain whether to risk all that has been gained. He has decided to wait awhile. Maybe a new drug will come along that will do the rest.

But he dreams of seeing her walk too. "Maybe we should try at least once more." What would you do?

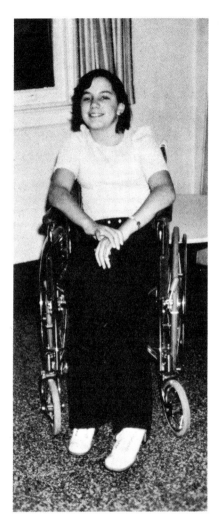